How to Get the Most Out of Rational Emotive Behaviour Therapy

How to Get the Most Out of Rational Emotive Behaviour Therapy: A Client's Guide is aimed at those who are either considering consulting or already seeing a Rational Emotive Behaviour Therapy (REBT) therapist.

This book is designed to help guide clients through the REBT process from before they start through to when they are looking towards an end of therapy and next steps. The goal is not to discuss specific REBT practice methods, but rather provide a comprehensive guide to topics such as:

- How to decide if REBT is right for you.
- How to prepare for your REBT session.
- Understanding the process of change in REBT.
- Learning to apply what you learn from REBT therapy sessions.

This concise and practical guide will help you to understand REBT, how to get the most out of each session and how you can ensure that you continue to benefit from it once therapy has ended.

Windy Dryden is in part-time clinical and consultative practice and is an international authority on REBT. He has worked in psychotherapy for more than 45 years and is the author and editor of over 285 books.

How to Get the Most Out of Rational Emotive Behaviour Therapy

A Client's Guide

Windy Dryden

R Routledge
Taylor & Francis Group

LONDON AND NEW YORK

First published 2025
by Routledge
4 Park Square, Milton Park, Abingdon, Oxon OX14 4RN

and by Routledge
605 Third Avenue, New York, NY 10158

Routledge is an imprint of the Taylor & Francis Group, an informa business

British Library Cataloguing-in-Publication Data
A catalogue record for this book is available from the British Library

ISBN: 9781032796475 (hbk)
ISBN: 9781032796000 (pbk)
ISBN: 9781003493198 (ebk)

DOI: 10.4324/9781003493198

Typeset in Times New Roman
by Newgen Publishing UK

Contents

Introduction

I have written this book for people who are either considering consulting a Rational Emotive Behaviour Therapy (REBT)
therapist or who are actually consulting such a therapist. You
can either read the book in one go or seek advice from a particular chapter or section that deals with an issue with which
you are currently concerned.

What This Book Does

I have written this book to help guide you through the REBT
process from the point at which you are trying to decide if REBT
is for you to the point where you have largely gone through the
process and are learning how to be your own therapist. In doing
so, I have discussed a variety of points of which I think REBT
clients should ideally be aware. These are, of course, personal,
and other REBT therapists would no doubt choose other points.
What lies behind my choice of points to discuss in this book is
not only my personal knowledge and experience as an REBT
therapist and a trainer of REBT therapists but also my knowledge of more general therapeutic issues and my willingness to
learn from practitioners of other approaches to therapy.

What This Book Does *Not* Do

What I have *not* done in this book is to discuss any specific
REBT methods that you can use to help you deal with your

DOI: 10.4324/9781003493198-1

problems or to take any specific REBT line. I have decided to take this stance because I do not want to interfere with the technical approach taken by your REBT therapist.

You may have been recommended to see a CBT therapist and then discovered that your therapist practises REBT. In my view, CBT is a psychotherapy tradition and not a specific psychotherapy approach. It is an umbrella term under which specific CBT approaches such as REBT can be placed. If you are confused about this please discuss it with your therapist.

Windy Dryden, February 2024
London, Eastbourne

Chapter 1

Decide if REBT Is for You

How is it that you have ended up either consulting or thinking of consulting an REBT therapist? How much do you know about REBT? Have you actively sought out an REBT therapist or were you recommended to do so? These are some of the questions that come to my mind as I invite you to decide whether or not REBT is for you. Indeed, these are some of the questions that I do ask people who come to see me, either to consult me as an REBT practitioner or to seek my help to determine which approach to therapy is best suited to them. Since I don't know your answers to these questions, let me deal with the issue of how you can best decide if REBT is for you in a more general way.

Common Factors That Span Different Psychotherapeutic Approaches

In the field of psychotherapy and counselling, it is recognized that different approaches have both common factors (i.e. common to all therapeutic approaches) and specific factors (i.e. specific to the particular approach under consideration). The main common factors include:

- The development and maintenance of an effective working alliance between you and your therapist.
- The provision of a safe space in which you can discuss whatever is important to you.

DOI: 10.4324/9781003493198-2

- The mobilization of hope whereby you come to see that you can effectively address your concerns.
- Experiencing your therapist as someone who is genuine with you, understands you and accepts you.

As I have said, these factors are common to all approaches to therapy and are not specific to REBT. While I have entitled this chapter 'Decide if REBT Is for You', when it comes to the presence or absence of these common factors, I suggest that your focus be more on deciding whether or not the *therapist* whom you have come to see is the right *person* for you to consult than on whether or not REBT is right for you. Thus, your therapist may be technically proficient in REBT, but if you don't feel safe talking to them about what really matters to you, you are right to have doubts about your therapist. Based on the above, here are some questions to ask yourself to help you make your decision about whether or not to work with your particular therapist:

- To what extent does my therapist understand my problems from my perspective?
- To what extent does my therapist accept me the way I am?
- To what extent is my therapist genuine in their interactions with me?
- To what extent do I feel safe to discuss what really matters to me with my therapist?
- To what extent does my therapist inspire hope in me that I can effectively deal with my problems?
- To what extent does my therapist foster a working relationship with me focused on dealing with my problems?

While it is unrealistic for your therapist to score top marks on all these points, they should score highly enough for you to consider working with them over time. If they score poorly on all these points, then, in all probability, they will not be able to help you much despite their proficiency in REBT. If the therapist scores highly on all but one or two points, then you should consider discussing your feelings with them on the points where they do not score highly. I will address the importance of discussing with your therapist matters to do with your therapy later in this book. For now, let me make two points.

First, if you don't feel able to discuss your concerns with your therapist, then this may, in itself, indicate that your therapist is not right for you.

Second, if you do decide to discuss your concerns with your therapist on these matters, the way your therapist responds is important. If they take your concerns seriously and respond without defensiveness, then these are good signs that you can work with the therapist and that you can deal with any rifts in your relationship that may occur over the course of therapy. However, if your therapist appears to dismiss your concerns and/or responds defensively, then this does not augur well for the future and you should consider finding yourself a different therapist.

Having made this point, don't forget that therapists are human too and may have their off days. However, if a therapist responds dismissively and or defensively more than once, then I do urge you to think very carefully about continuing to work with that person.

REBT's Main Specific Factors

In making a decision concerning REBT's suitability for you, it is important for you to understand some of the therapy's main features. I made the point in the introduction that REBT is a specific approach that comes under the umbrella of the CBT tradition. Having said that, let me outline some of REBT's main specific factors.

REBT Focuses on the Way You Think and Act in the Context of Your Emotions and in the Situations in Which You Experience These Emotions

REBT stands for 'Rational Emotive Behaviour Therapy', but as this approach falls under the CBT tradition, you should expect that therapy will focus on your behaviour and thinking as well as your emotions.

Focus on Behaviour

Let's start with behaviour, as this is the easiest of the two terms to grasp. Your REBT therapist will focus a lot on the ways in which you behave, particularly in situations in which you experience your problem(s). However, your REBT therapist may also be interested to understand what may be termed 'action tendencies'. These describe situations in which you feel an urge to act in a certain way but don't actually do so. Such action tendencies are particularly valuable in helping your therapist discover your hard-to-identify emotions (such as envy and hurt). Understanding the difference between an action tendency and an overt behaviour may also help you see that you don't have to act on your action tendency, which is particularly important with problems of anger and self-discipline.

The focus on behaviour in REBT is particularly linked to an understanding of your goals and values. Thus, expect your REBT therapist to enquire about the extent to which your problem-related behaviour helps you to meet your goals and to what extent it is consistent with your personally held values. Consequently, during therapy, you can expect your therapist to encourage you to act in ways that help you to achieve your goals and are consistent with your values as well as to help you to identify, reflect on and deal with obstacles to the execution of such behaviour.

A particular focus on behaviour that your therapist may well take, particularly if you have problems with anxiety, is to consider your use of safety behaviours (i.e. behaviours which you use to keep yourself safe from threat but in ways that *may* serve to maintain your anxiety problems). REBT practice is strongly underpinned by research in CBT; while studies in the past showed the negative effects of such safety behaviours, more recent studies have shown that they may be useful in encouraging you to face your fears. Effective REBT therapists keep abreast of the research literature and modify their practice accordingly.

Focus on Thinking

In REBT, there will also be a focus on thinking as this has a strong bearing on how you feel and act. While there are different types of thinking, your REBT therapist will help you to focus mainly on the rigid and extreme attitudes that REBT says lie at the core of your emotional and behavioural problems. In addition, sometimes the focus will be on the inferences or interpretations that you make in problem-related situations. However, it is likely that your REBT therapist will first encourage you to assume temporarily that your inferences are correct so that they can help you pinpoint the rigid and extreme attitudes that from an REBT perspective explain the presence of your problems. Your therapist will provide you with examples so that you fully understand this principle. If you do not understand, please let your therapist know this and they will help clarify any points.

REBT Focuses on How You Unwittingly Maintain Your Problems Rather Than on How They Originally Began. Consequently, REBT Focuses on What You Can Do Now to Address Your Problems

It is often thought that REBT therapists are not interested in your past. This is not correct, and in REBT you may talk about whatever it is you are bothered about, be it your past, your present or your future. Having said this, REBT therapists tend not to believe that helping you to understand the past roots of your present problems will be curative in the long term without you doing something about these problems in the present. REBT therapists generally hold to the view that relevant past experiences may have contributed to your current problems but do not account fully for these problems. REBT therapists explain this by pointing out that if 100 people all experienced exactly the same adversities in the past as you, not all of them would have developed the same problems as you. Some may have developed other problems, and others would not have developed problems at all. Rather, it is the attitudes that you developed from these experiences and still hold currently that largely account for your problems together with the behaviour that stems from these views.

For example, take the problem of jealousy. If you have such a problem, it may well be the case that you felt jealous of your sibling as a child. However, this insight will not help you if you continue to act in jealous ways in the present (e.g. by preventing your partner from doing things, checking on their whereabouts). Such behaviour will reinforce and strengthen the rigid and extreme attitudes that underpin your jealous feelings and will nullify any effect that insight into the possible roots of your problem might have. As a result, unless your REBT therapist helps you to deal with the ways in which you currently, but unwittingly, maintain your problem, then it is unlikely that you will gain much long-term benefit from therapy.

REBT Focuses on Helping You to Put into Practice Between Sessions What You Learn in Sessions

When you consult an REBT therapist, it is unlikely that you will derive any benefit unless you learn something in the therapy sessions. However, such learning is likely to be academic and thus of limited value to you unless you put it into practice between therapy sessions. Consequently, in REBT, expect your therapist to negotiate with you on ways of implementing your session-derived insights into relevant situations in your everyday life. The extent to which you do so will determine how much you get from REBT. Thus, I am often asked whether REBT is helpful. What is my answer? Yes, if you use it; no, if you don't! I will discuss the issue of applying what you learn in Chapter 6.

REBT Focuses on Helping You to Become Your Own REBT Therapist

While all approaches to counselling and psychotherapy have as an aim you learning how to help yourself in the future after therapy has ended, REBT therapists, more than other practitioners, implement this aim in specific ways. They do this by teaching their clients REBT self-help skills throughout the therapy process. Thus, your therapist will use an REBT-related framework to teach you how to assess your own problematic thinking, feeling and behaviour in problem-related episodes and how to respond productively to these situations. You will then be encouraged to use this framework for yourself between sessions and helped to refine your developing skills in subsequent sessions by your therapist when you report back on how you implemented your skills. Given this emphasis on helping you to become your own REBT therapist, it is likely that your therapist will give you increasing responsibility to help yourself as therapy progresses. They will do this by gradually fading their own active contribution to the process, becoming more of a consultant and giving you feedback on your developing self-helping skills rather than actively taking the lead as they did at the beginning of therapy.

Because REBT emphasizes teaching clients self-help skills, there are a number of REBT-oriented workbooks available that can be used as an adjunct to therapy. Your therapist may suggest incorporating such a workbook into your therapy. While some clients value using such workbooks, others find them too for-mulaic and would prefer not to use them.

Flexible REBT therapists will be mindful of the fact that while REBT does emphasize the teaching of self-help skills as an integral part of the therapy, some clients do not want to learn these skills in such a deliberate manner. These flexible therapists adjust REBT accordingly. I will discuss the issue of becoming your own REBT therapist more fully in Chapter 8.

In this chapter, I have set out to give you a flavour of some of REBT's distinctive features. I have also stressed that, as REBT values explicitness, it is very likely that your therapist will make clear to you how they will use REBT to understand and deal with your problems. Thus, it should be easier for you to judge whether or not REBT is for you than it would be if you were consulting a therapist who practises a non-CBT approach. If you are still in doubt, most REBT therapists will suggest a brief 'trial period' of therapy where you can experience REBT for yourself as a way of judging whether or not you wish to make a firm commitment to becoming an REBT client.

In addition, some therapists will send prospective clients a brief description of REBT so that they can see if it is an approach that they may be interested in. An example of such a description is found in Appendix 1. Ask your prospective REBT therapist if they have such a brief description they can send you.

If you have decided that REBT is for you and you have found a properly trained therapist to work with, you will need to make a number of practical agreements with them to ensure that therapy gets off on the right foot. This will be the subject of the next chapter.

Chapter 2

Make Practical Agreements with Your Therapist

Therapy, of whatever type, works better if the two involved parties, namely you and your therapist, agree on a number of important points. These points can be placed in one of two realms: the practical realm of REBT and the therapeutic realm of REBT.

The practical realm of REBT involves such matters as your therapist's fee, if one is charged, and how it is to be paid; how frequently the two of you will meet; how many sessions you will have; and what the cancellation policy of your therapist is. If your therapist works in a clinic, then there may well be additional practical issues to be discussed and agreed. I will deal with such practical agreements in this chapter.

The therapeutic realm of REBT involves such matters as how you and your therapist see your problems and what your respective goals are in regard to these problems. It also involves understanding what steps you are both going to take to address your problems and help you achieve your goals and the commitment you are prepared to make with respect to carrying out these steps. I will deal with such therapeutic agreements in the next chapter.

While the distinction between the practical and therapeutic realm of REBT is somewhat arbitrary – after all, how you and your therapist negotiate on the practical issues may either be therapeutic or non-therapeutic – it is a useful way of separating out issues concerning why you have come for therapy and what

DOI: 10.4324/9781003493198-3

you want to achieve (i.e. the therapeutic realm) and issues that are designed to grease the wheels for both of you (i.e. the practical realm) as you both strive to achieve your goals. So here are some of the practical agreements you will need to make with your REBT therapist.

The Length of Therapy Sessions

One of the practical aspects of your therapy that your therapist should make clear at the outset is the length of therapy sessions. Actually, when most therapists talk about therapy 'sessions', they most often refer to the therapeutic hour as lasting 50 minutes rather than a full hour. The tradition of the 50-minute therapeutic hour has come about to reflect the fact that therapists need to take a short break between sessions for several reasons, most typically to write notes, clear their head, go to the toilet or make and/or take phone calls. If your therapist operates a 50-minute hour practice, then they should make this clear to you. Otherwise, you may think that your sessions last for 60 minutes and may consider that you have been short-changed if your therapist stops sessions after 50 minutes without explanation. If your therapist does not make this clear, then, by all means, ask them. Sometimes therapy sessions may be shorter or longer, and if any changes are made to an established and agreed arrangement with respect to the length of therapy sessions, then this needs to be fully discussed, understood by you and your therapist, and agreed to by both of you. Any changes to an established session length may result in pro rata changes to any fees that are being charged (see the next section).

The Fee

If you are seeing your REBT therapist in a National Health Service (NHS) clinic or facility or in an organization that does not levy a fee, then what I have to say does not concern you, although if this is the case it is very likely that the number of sessions you can agree to have with your therapist will be limited (see the section, The Total Number of REBT Sessions, later in the chapter). However, if it is the case that your therapist levies a fee, then it is very important that you understand what this fee is. I have known clients who have not enquired about the therapist's fees and have had quite a shock when they received the latter's invoice because the therapist, in these cases, had not told the clients what their fees were. So please do ask your therapist what their fee is if they do not venture this information themself. I suggest that you do this on initial enquiry to save time. If your therapist's fees are out of your financial reach, it is useful to enquire about whether they have a sliding scale, but if not or if the reduced fee is still out of your range, then it is useful to ask the therapist if they have a colleague whose fees are within your range. Be prepared, therefore, to tell the referring therapist how much you are prepared to pay.

You may well be thinking that how much you can afford per therapy session will be based on how many sessions you need, but please bear in mind that therapists cannot tell their prospective clients how many sessions they may need until they have carried out a thorough assessment.

When you and your therapist have agreed to a fee, it is useful to discover if the fee (or part of it) will be levied if you contact and discuss matters with the therapist between sessions or if a fee will be charged for other matters. For example, I once saw a client for individual REBT who at the same time was having couples therapy with a different therapist. The client had to be hospitalized but requested a couples therapy session with her couples therapist while she was in hospital. The couples therapist came to the hospital and duly conducted the session. To my client's surprise and consternation, the therapist billed the couple for three hours as opposed to the usual one-hour charge for the session. When questioned, the therapist told the couple that he was billing them for the one-hour session and the two hours that he gave up to travel to and from the hospital to carry out the session. The point that I wish to make here does not concern the rights and wrongs of charging for two hours' travel time but concerns the fact that the therapist did not make clear that he was going to do this in advance of agreeing to carry out the hospital-based therapy session. Also, the client couple could have asked if there was going to be an additional charge, as the therapist would have to make the journey out of his professional time. This failure to make an agreement about the additional charge, which I argue is in the practical realm of therapy, had quite an adverse effect on the therapeutic relationship and it took quite a while for the therapist to regain the couple's trust in him.

The Cancellation Policy

When you contract with your REBT therapist and if they do levy a fee, then it is important that you understand what their cancellation policy is. Once you understand this, you may wish to suggest amendments based on your unique circumstances. This should lead to a discussion and hopefully to a mutually agreed policy. Possible ambiguities of the terms of the policy should be highlighted by one or both parties and clarified. For example, I have a 48-hour cancellation policy, which, as I point out to prospective clients, is different from one specifying two days. Thus, if a client and I have scheduled for, say, 11am on Wednesday and they wish to cancel it without paying my fee, then they need to inform me of that by 11am on the Monday before. If they cancel their appointment at 12 noon on Monday, they will be charged, since they have not given me the full 48 hours' notice.

Some therapists will not charge a fee if you cancel your session without giving full notice if you become ill or a member of your family becomes ill, for example, while others will still levy their fee under these circumstances. It is important that your therapist is clear with you about the exceptions they are prepared to make concerning fee payment when you have not given full notice, and if they do not do this, then, in my view, you should ask them.

Some therapists apply their cancellation policy to themselves, while others don't. For example, if I have to cancel a client's session and I have not given them 48 hours' notice, then their next scheduled session is provided free of charge. Again, the therapist should ideally make this explicit to you as their client.

The Total Number of REBT Sessions

If you are thinking about consulting an REBT therapist, it is likely that you are wondering how many sessions you are likely to need. However, while this is a reasonable question to ask your therapist, it is important for you to realize that the number of sessions you will need cannot be validly determined by your therapist when you first contact them and give very rudimentary information about yourself and your problems. As I have stated previously, it can only be answered after your therapist has met with you and carried out a full assessment of your problems and what you want to achieve from therapy. Having said that, here is what I say to prospective clients:

The length of therapy depends on how many problems you have, what you want to achieve with respect to these problems, how chronic your problems are and how hard you work in therapy. So, if you have a few problems that are acute in nature, are prepared to work hard to address these problems in between therapy sessions and to work towards achievable, specific goals, then therapy is likely to be short-term in nature. However, if you have a large number of problems that are chronic in nature, you think that change will occur in therapy sessions rather than by what you do between sessions and your goals are vague, then therapy is likely to be longer term.

The Frequency of REBT Sessions

Normally, you will see your REBT therapist once a week until you make progress, and then sessions are likely to be spaced out more. This is because a major goal of REBT is for you to become your own therapist, as I mentioned in Chapter 1 and as I will discuss more fully in Chapter 8. As you learn the skills of REBT, you will be encouraged to take increasing responsibility for applying them in your life, and the increasing spacing out of therapy sessions helps you to do that.

There may be times when you may see your therapist more than once a week. This may reflect the complexity of your problems or that you are going through a crisis; both of these situations indicate that you need more therapeutic input than weekly sessions. However, even under these conditions, you will be encouraged to take responsibility for dealing with these issues as far as you are able and to reduce the frequency of sessions when you are ready to do so. This readiness will be assessed by you and your therapist together.

Confidentiality

You may think that the contact between you and your REBT therapist is completely confidential, but in reality, this is unlikely to be the case. Here is a list of situations where your therapist may reveal information about you or take action without your permission:

- When mandated to do so by the court.
- To protect your well-being when you are not able or willing to do so.
- To protect the well-being of others when you pose a threat to them without yourself taking steps to protect them.

• If you steadfastly refuse to pay your therapist's fees so that they have to take legal action to be paid.

Your therapist may have additional exceptions to complete confidentiality, and if so, they should inform you about these. This latter point is the main one that I wish to stress. One of the ethical principles that counselling and psychotherapy is based on is known as *informed consent*. From your perspective as a client, this means that you need to be clearly informed about something before you can properly consent to it. Because one of the features of REBT is its explicitness, its practitioners should, ideally, make explicit all the exceptions to complete confidentiality. However, should this not happen, take responsibility and ask your therapist directly.

The Form of the Contract

So far, in this chapter, I have focused on the practical agreements that you need to make with your therapist if you are to get the most out of REBT. While the important point is that these agreements should be made, you and your therapist need to determine together the form that they will take. Thus, such agreements may be made informally or formally.

An informally made agreement tends to be verbal and as such it is open to misinterpretation and misunderstanding. Thus, earlier I mentioned that I have a 48-hour cancellation policy. If I explain what this means verbally, the client may not understand what I have said or forget the nature of the policy. This may lead to problems later when the client fails to give the stated notice and questions why they must pay for the cancelled session.

A formally made agreement tends to be written and may even be signed by both parties. While such an agreement is not open to misinterpretation or misunderstanding, it may well put off some clients who complain that it is too businesslike and indicates that the therapist does not trust the client. In Appendix 2, you will find an example of a formal agreement.

My point here is to state the importance of you and your therapist agreeing to the form of the contract that you have decided to make in light of the fact that both approaches have advantages and disadvantages.

Having dealt with the practical agreements that you will need to make with your REBT therapist, I now, in the next chapter, consider the therapeutic agreements you will need to make with them.

Chapter 3

Make Therapeutic Agreements with Your Therapist

In the previous chapter, I discussed a number of practical agreements that it is important for you to make with your REBT therapist if your working relationship with them is going to get off on the right foot and stay that way. However, most of these practical agreements are common to most, if not all, approaches to therapy and are certainly not unique to REBT. In this chapter, I am going to focus on the therapeutic agreements you need to make with your REBT therapist that do pertain to REBT and concern why you have come for therapy: to address your emotional problems and get on with the business of living.

While clients who are seeing non-REBT therapists will make similar agreements, I will concentrate here on agreements that typify REBT. As I have already mentioned, one of the features of REBT that characterizes this therapeutic approach is its emphasis on explicitness. This means that you can expect your REBT practitioner to spell out what they mean about a number of important issues, as we shall see. If you think that your REBT therapist is not being clear about something, then ask them. They should tell you. If not, they should tell you why they are not prepared to tell you. The distinct advantage of therapist explicitness is that it enables you to understand where your therapist is coming from and to agree or disagree with the explicitly expressed points they have made. In this chapter, I will discuss the nature of the therapeutic agreements that you need to make with your therapist that ideally are very much facilitated

DOI: 10.4324/9781003493198-4

by their explicit style of communication. Later in this chapter, I will discuss the importance of speaking up if there is anything you don't understand about what your therapist is saying, if you disagree with anything that they say or if you find anything that they say or do unhelpful.

The Nature of Therapeutic Agreements

In this section I will discuss six different types of therapeutic agreements you need to make with your therapist. While your agreement on some points may be more explicit than on others, for REBT to be fully effective you need to have clear agreement on all six points.

Agreements about Your Problem(s)

You have probably come to REBT because you have one or more emotional or behavioural problems for which you are seeking help. It is important that your therapist listens carefully to these problems, communicates that they understand how you see these problems from your frame of reference and acknowledges that you want to address them. Later, they will, in all probability, offer you an REBT-based understanding of these problems, but at the outset, it is important that you agree with them on which problems you wish to address. Some therapists will introduce you to the idea of a problem list on which you put, in writing, what problems you want to cover in therapy. Please bear in mind that this list is not set in stone, and you may add to it or subtract from it over the course of therapy.

Generally, only problems that are within your control to tackle should be on the list and those that are outside your control should not be included.

Alan was having problems with his partner and was very angry with her because she was very untidy around the house; Alan responded to this by yelling at her. When his therapist asked Alan what his problem was, he said it was his partner's untidiness. Alan's REBT therapist explained to Alan why she did not want to put this on Alan's problem list. The therapist helped Alan see that his partner's untidy behaviour was under her control rather than his. Alan came to see that what was under his control were his feelings (unhealthy anger) and his behaviour (yelling). As Alan's feelings of unhealthy anger and yelling behaviour were unlikely to help him effectively address his partner's untidiness with her, his therapist invited him to regard his feelings and behaviour as problematic in this context and thus to put his response to her untidiness on the problem list rather than the untidiness itself.

Generally, only emotional and/or behavioural problems should be put on the problem list and not practical problems. Thus, if you are experiencing financial problems in your life, then this, on its own, is not a matter that can be directly dealt with by REBT. Rather, you need to consult a debt counsellor or financial adviser for such practical problems. However, you may also have emotional problems about these practical, financial problems and these emotional problems can be tackled with REBT. They may, with your assent, be placed on your problem list.

Agreements about Goals

For every problem that you are seeking help for, it is useful to have as clear an idea as you can of what you want to achieve by addressing it with your REBT therapist. I usually explain the importance of goals like this:

Imagine that you go to a railway terminus and say to the person selling tickets, 'I don't want to go to Brighton'. This person will either be at a loss as to what to do or will sell you a ticket for anywhere that is not Brighton. In either case, you are likely to be unhappy with the result. In the same way as expressing clearly where you want to go to a train ticket seller, doing the same thing with your REBT therapist will aid both of you to collaborate on working towards achieving your therapeutic goals.

To help you with goal setting, your REBT therapist may use the acronym 'SMART' to indicate the criteria for clearly formulated goals. Here is what each letter stands for:

- *S* stands for 'specific'. The more specific you can be about your goals, the more you will be able to see how to achieve them. Thus, goals such as 'I want to be happy', while laudable, are very vague and, as such, will be difficult to achieve. On the other hand, 'I want to deal with the prospect of criticism with healthy concern rather than anxiety and approach people who I think may criticise me rather than avoid them' is a clearly expressed goal and its specificity will help you achieve it.
- *M* stands for 'measurable'. The more you can measure your progress towards your goal, the more likely it is that you will persist in taking steps to achieve it. For example, the goal 'I want to tidy my house' is difficult to measure, whereas the goal 'I want to spend one hour a day tidying my house' is measurable and you can track your progress towards achieving it.
- *A* stands for 'attainable'. It is important to set goals that can actually be achieved by you. Thus, the goal 'I want to be free from anxiety' is probably unachievable, whereas the goal 'I want to respond to feeling anxious by working towards feeling healthy concern' is achievable.
- *R* stands for 'realistic'. You may set a goal that is attainable (e.g. 'I want to exercise in the gym for an hour a day'), but it

may not be realistic for you to achieve it. For example, you may live very far from a gym, and your work and family commitments may be too onerous for you to achieve this goal. While it is attainable in the sense that you have the ability to do it, it is not realistic in that you cannot find the time to do it. By contrast, 'exercising for twenty minutes a day by running around the nearby park' may be both attainable and realistic.

- *T* stands for 'time-bound'. It is important for you to set a time frame for achieving your goal. If you do not do this, you may be tempted to keep postponing working towards achieving it. Thus, compare 'I want to write my paper' with 'I want to write my paper by the end of this month'. While it is important to give yourself a specific time frame to achieve your goal, ensure that this frame is realistic and gives you some margin for error.

While your REBT therapist will keep the concept of SMART goals in mind when working with you, they will not try to impose it on you in a slavish manner. As I stress throughout this book, competent REBT therapists are flexible, and while they may think that encouraging you to develop SMART goals is the best way of helping you to get the most out of REBT, they also recognize that you may not find the development of such goals helpful, or your problems may not lend themselves to such an approach to goal formulation. In such cases, you and your therapist should ideally strive to formulate goals that make sense to both of you. You and your therapist may need to engage in some negotiation over this point, but a jointly agreed goal is more likely to be achieved than one that is either imposed on you or one that your therapist has serious reservations about.

Before leaving the topic of goals, I want to make one other important point. You are more likely to achieve your goals if you are prepared to commit yourself to achieving them and to accept the sacrifices that goal pursuit inevitably involves.

Two friends, John and Jack, struggle with procrastination and are falling behind in their studies as a result. Both want to begin key essays and do sustained work on them so they can submit them on or before the deadline. John is committed to achieving this goal and is prepared to tolerate not attending a number of social events that he would like to attend in order to achieve it. In other words, he is willing to put up with the sacrifices that working towards achieving his goal would entail. Jack is also committed to achieving his goal but, unlike John, is not prepared to miss out on attending the same social events. In other words, Jack is not willing to put up with the sacrifices that pursuing his goal would entail. Who is more likely to achieve his goals, John or Jack? The answer is, of course, John.

Agreements about the REBT Focus

An idea that is widespread about therapy in general is that when you go to see a therapist, you spend a lot of time talking about the past roots of your problems rather than about your problems as they exist in the present. The idea here is that if you understand how you acquired your problems in the first place, this will help you to address them in the present. However, REBT has attracted the opposing viewpoint: that when you go to see an REBT therapist, you talk about the present and the future but not about the past, and you focus on how you unwittingly maintain your problems rather than on how you originally acquired them. While there is an element of truth about this latter view, it is not quite accurate. First of all, your REBT therapist will encourage you to talk about whatever you are troubled about. So, if you are preoccupied with events in the past, then your therapist will help you to talk about them. Having said that, while REBT therapists recognize that your past experiences contribute to your present problems, they also argue that your current rigid and extreme attitudes towards these experiences play a large role in why your problems persist.

So, while you will be allowed to discuss whatever you are preoccupied with in REBT and while due weight will be given to the influence of the past on the present, a distinctive feature of REBT is that a clear focus will be placed on your current attitudes and how you currently behave as a way of helping you to address your problems effectively. If you cannot agree on such a focus with your REBT therapist, then REBT may not be the right therapy of choice for you. If this turns out to be the case, your therapist will discuss with you a judicious referral to a therapist who practises an approach that better meets your ideas on the issue of what to focus on in therapy.

Agreements about the Therapist and Client Roles

I sometimes hear it said about therapy that it is a process that involves you talking and your therapist 'sorting you out'. This is very much at variance with what role your therapist plays and what role you are expected to play in REBT. Most REBT therapists view the therapeutic relationship as collaborative, which means that you work together in the service of your psychological health. However, both parties bring different resources to this collaboration, and in this section I will outline what these resources are. Collectively, these resources add up to your respective roles.

Your Therapist's Role in REBT

Here is a list of what I consider to be your REBT therapist's responsibilities in REBT, which taken together constitute their role.

1. To bring their REBT knowledge to bear on the assessment and formulation of your problems and to communicate this clearly and explicitly.

2. To suggest and explain ways of tackling your problems and to make clear how these relate to the assessment/formulation and how they will help you achieve your goals.
3. To engage you as an active participant in a collaborative relationship where you work together in the service of your therapeutic goals
4. To identify and respond to anything that you are unclear about or have reservations about in the therapeutic process.
5. To identify potential and actual obstacles to goal achievement and to deal with these in a sensitive way.
6. To ask for feedback about the therapeutic process and discuss your suggestions for modifications to your therapy.

Your Role as Client in REBT

Here is a list of what I consider to be your responsibilities in REBT as a client, which taken together constitute your role.

1. To speak openly about your problems, but to do so in a way and at a rate that is helpful for you.
2. To be active in the therapeutic process; to speak up and give your opinion about salient aspects of the therapy.

You might think that, as your REBT therapist is the expert in REBT, they should know what they are doing and, thus, that if you don't understand a point they are making then that is your fault. Fortunately, this is a misguided view. It is misguided for a number of reasons.

First, it assumes that your REBT therapist can do no wrong. Since your REBT therapist is human first and a therapist a distant second, they are susceptible to all the vagaries of being human. In other words, they are fallible and can make mistakes and get things wrong. Even the most skilful and experienced REBT therapist may, for example, explain something in a manner that you just don't understand.

Second, if you assume that your therapist is infallible and always explains things in an understandable way, then it must be your fault if you don't understand a point that they make. The consequence of this view is that you are mainly in therapy to be the passive recipient of your therapist's wisdom and that if you don't understand something, then there is no point in bringing this to their attention since the fault lies in you. Again, the reality is very different. REBT is a collaborative enterprise, and you and your therapist are equal participants in the therapeutic process. As you are both fallible, you both can get things wrong, and the best way that human beings have of putting things right is to communicate about them. Let's see what this means in practice.

Fiona was seeing an REBT therapist about her performance anxiety. Her therapist assessed her problem and suggested a way of dealing with it which Fiona only understood in part. Her therapist assumed that Fiona understood fully his formulation and treatment suggestions and proceeded accordingly.

Fiona has two basic options here. First, she could say nothing and hope that she will understand more fully later her therapist's conceptualization of her problem and how she can best deal with it. Second, she could speak up and tell her therapist that she does not understand.

I strongly suggest that she do the latter. Here is how she might address the issue with her therapist:

Fiona: I'm not clear why you think that me doing what you call 'over-preparing' my talk is a problem. Can you explain what you mean, please?

Once the therapist re-explained her point, Fiona was not entirely convinced.

Fiona: Well, I kind of see what you mean, but your suggestion that I limit my preparation to an hour a day is not something I am prepared to do. I'll limit it, but not to an hour a day.

You can see from this brief vignette that Fiona is showing herself to be a full participant in the therapy process, speaking up when she does not understand something or does not agree with something. In this way she is discharging her responsibility as a client.

While REBT therapists value such therapist–client collaboration, they cannot check every point with their clients, so they rely to some extent on their clients speaking up and telling them when they don't understand something, don't agree with something or think that their therapists have got things wrong. If you don't speak up as a client, you will increase the chances that 'obstacles to client change' will occur in therapy, which means that you will not make expected progress because in some way you silently have not signed on to certain key therapeutic points with which your therapist thought you agreed. I will discuss this issue in the context of dealing with lack of progress in Chapter 7.

3. To undertake to carry out agreed tasks in the service of your goals (discussed in the next section and Chapter 6) and to be open about reasons why you did not do the tasks if this was the case.

If it transpires that there is not a good enough match between the therapist and client roles as outlined here that you think will be helpful to you in therapy, then it is important to discuss this discrepancy with your therapist and decide together what is the best way forward. If such an agreement about both of your roles cannot be made, then therapeutic progress will be severely compromised and you may be better off seeking help from a therapist who practises an approach which better approximates your views on such roles.

Agreements about Therapeutic Tasks

REBT involves you and your therapist doing various things in therapy sessions and you doing things between therapy sessions to help you achieve your therapeutic goals. For the purposes of this discussion, I will refer to these as therapeutic tasks. Note well my point that both you and your therapist are expected to carry out such tasks in REBT. What kind of agreements do you and your therapist need to make about tasks in REBT, whether you do so explicitly or implicitly? Here are some of the main agreements that you and your therapist need to make with respect to therapeutic tasks:

- That you both understand what your respective tasks are and agree to implement them in the course of therapy.
- That you both understand how carrying out your respective tasks will help you to achieve your therapeutic goals as a client.
- That you both understand what your skills and capabilities are as a client to carry out your therapeutic tasks and are both prepared to take the necessary steps to help you to implement these tasks if you cannot do so.
- That you both agree to make modifications to your respective tasks should it become necessary to do so.
- That you both understand that your therapist will teach you how to implement your tasks outside of therapy sessions, and the more you are able to do this, the more they will encourage you to take increasing responsibility to become your own therapist.

Agreements about Ending

I mentioned in the previous section that one of the issues that you and your therapist need to agree on is when you will take increasing responsibility in therapy to become your own therapist. When this occurs, then you need to discuss how you are going to end the process. There are a number of approaches to ending therapy in a planned way:

- Meet regularly (say weekly) and then set a date for the final session. A review session or sessions may or may not be scheduled.
- Decrease the frequency between sessions before setting a date for the final session. Again, a review session or sessions may or may not be scheduled.
- Decrease the frequency between sessions without setting a final date so that there are very long gaps between sessions, which effectively serve as review sessions.

Here as elsewhere, the important issue is that you agree with your therapist on the best way to end the process for your own particular situation.

In the next chapter, I discuss what you can do to prepare yourself for therapy sessions so that you may derive the most benefit from them.

Chapter 4

Prepare for Your REBT Sessions

You may think that now that you are in therapy, all you need to do is to turn up for your therapy sessions and talk. After all, isn't therapy supposed to be the talking cure? Well, yes and no! Obviously, you need to talk about what you are bothered about in your life, but one way to get the most out of therapy based on the principles of REBT is to come prepared for your therapy sessions.

What preparations you might make will, of course, depend on what problems you wish to discuss and the phase of therapy you are in. However, you might find the following guidelines helpful.

Develop a Problem and Goal List

Develop a Problem List

Before you attend your first therapy session, or as soon as possible after this session, I suggest that you make a list of the problems you want to address in therapy. This is known as a 'problem list'. Make sure that the problems on this list are those that *you* think that you have and that *you* want to address rather than problems that others think you have and want you to address in therapy. At this point, I suggest that you phrase these problems in your own words. If necessary, your therapist will help you to reword your problems so that they are expressed in a form that will best help you to tackle them. This normally

DOI: 10.4324/9781003493198-5

involves you and your therapist working to phrase your problems as clearly and specifically as possible.

As mentioned in the previous chapter, REBT works best if you address problems that are within your direct control to change.

Develop a Goal List

I also suggest that you develop a companion list of what *you* want to achieve from therapy with respect to these problems. So, for every problem you have listed, see if you can set a goal. As you set your goals, bear in mind that the presence of a healthy state is easier to achieve than the reduction or absence of a negative state. Thus, the goal 'I want to feel concerned about the possibility of being rejected' is easier to achieve than 'I don't want to feel anxious about the possibility of being rejected'.

Again, put your goals into your own words and your therapist will, if necessary, help you to express them in a form that will best help you to achieve them. Please remember one important point about therapy goals, though. You probably won't achieve them fully. As Marilyn Grey once said: 'No one ever has it "all together". That's like trying to eat once and for all.'

The same point that I made concerning nominating problems that are within your direct control to change also applies to the topic of goals. The more your goals are within your power to achieve, the more likely it is that you will achieve them.

Come with a Clear Idea of What You Want to Discuss in Each Therapy Session

You have met your therapist and had an opportunity to tell them why you are seeking help, and you have decided to work together. You could just turn up for subsequent therapy sessions without doing any preparation but, in my view, you would not get as much out of these sessions as you would do if you came with a clear idea of what you want to discuss. Such preparation can take a number of different forms, of which the following is a sample:

- Keep a log of events that you found upsetting in the week preceding your therapy session, perhaps putting these events in some kind of order in which you want to discuss them.
- Select a problem from your problem list that you want to address (known as the 'nominated problem') and choose a specific example of that problem to discuss with your therapist.
- Take a specific example of your nominated problem or a specific event about which you were upset and try to make sense of it using REBT's *ABC* framework that your therapist outlined to you or developed with you.
- Bring to the session anything that you want to revisit or did not understand from the previous session or sessions. This is an important point that I will address more fully in due course.

Session Agenda

Now, your REBT therapist may well suggest that you develop an agenda for each therapy session that you attend. The purpose of this agenda is for you and your therapist to ensure that you cover what you both want to deal with in the session and for you both to use session time effectively. In addition to the items mentioned in the previous section, agenda items for which you can prepare beforehand include:

- One or more inventories that provide your therapist with an objective guide to how your mood is changing as a result of therapy (which may be completed just before your session, to save therapy time).

- A review of any between-session activities you have agreed to do (discussed more fully in Chapter 6).

The important thing about the session agenda is that you and your therapist use it flexibly, not rigidly. So, if something really important comes up in a session that is not on the agenda, you should have the freedom to explore it rather than have it ruled 'off limits' because it does not feature on the agenda.

Matters Arising

While I am not suggesting that an REBT session should be likened to a business meeting, if one is to set an agenda for therapy sessions, then it makes sense to have an item on that agenda entitled 'matters arising'. This means that you should bring to the session anything that emerged from the previous session or the intervening period that you wish to discuss. This might include:

- Anything you did not understand from the previous session.
- Anything you disagreed with from the previous session.
- Any doubts, reservations or objections you had about the previous session or about therapy in general.

I will discuss this issue more fully in Chapter 7. In the next chapter, however, I will outline a process view of REBT so you can see how your therapy is likely to unfold.

Chapter 5

Understand the Process of Change

You may find it helpful to have some idea of the process of change in REBT so that you can anticipate the process that lies ahead. As such, I am going to outline a number of stages that you may go through as you make progress on the problems for which you have sought REBT. I want to make clear at the outset that I am not putting forward these stages as those you *must* go through and I am not suggesting that the order in which I present them is the only or the correct order. Rather, you should regard them as stages that you *may* go through, albeit perhaps in a different order.

Stage 1: Admitting That You Have a Problem (or Problems) and Accepting Yourself for Having It (or Them)

While most people who seek REBT do so because they recognize that they have a problem, this is not universally the case. Thus, you may have been sent for help or are consulting an REBT therapist because you consider that you have to, for some reason, rather than you want to do so. Indeed, you may feel ambivalent about seeking help: part of you wants to, while another part of you does not. It is important that you be honest with your REBT therapist about where you are on this issue so that they can help themself and you discover whether or not you have a problem, and if so, what might be stopping you from admitting to having it.

DOI: 10.4324/9781003493198-6

One of the major blocks to admitting that you have a problem is a sense of shame. Here you believe something like: 'If I admit that I have this problem, then it would mean that I am weak, inadequate and worthless.' If this applies to you, then your therapist will help you to address this self-devaluation attitude before moving on to helping you to deal with the problem about which you feel ashamed.

You may also devalue yourself even though you are readily able to admit to having a problem (which I refer to here as a primary problem). While this 'meta-problem' needs addressing at some point, once you have disclosed it to your therapist they will help you to determine whether it needs therapeutic attention before you address your primary problem or after you have done so. Basically, the more your meta-problem interferes with you focusing your attention on your primary problem, either in therapy sessions or between them, the more likely it is that you and your therapist need to address your meta-problem before your primary problem. However, here as elsewhere in the therapy process, such decisions are made jointly between you and your therapist rather than unilaterally by your therapist.

Stage 2: Understanding Your Problems: Assessment and Formulation

Some REBT therapists prefer to have an idea of all the problems for which you are seeking help and to understand the connections between them before helping you to tackle these problems one at a time. This is known as a case formulation. This formulation helps your therapist to plan therapy based on an overall understanding of your problems and the mechanisms that are at play in their inter-connections. Your therapist will not do this without your active participation, and perhaps the most important thing about a case formulation is that it is arrived at jointly between you and your therapist. This approach may be regarded as a formulation-based approach to REBT.

Other REBT therapists will prefer to begin therapy by focusing on the problem you want to start with and will wait to discover the connections among your problems later. This approach may be regarded as a problem-based approach to REBT. In this approach, the therapist will help you and themself understand the dynamics of the problem that you have selected to tackle first. This is known as problem assessment. Again, you will be expected to take an active role in problem assessment, providing relevant information and agreeing on the assessment which you arrive at jointly.

You will see that the therapist carries out problem assessment and a case formulation in both approaches but the order in which they do this is different in each.

In my experience, most REBT therapists adopt a problem-based approach rather than a formulation-based approach to REBT. This stems from the view of the founder of REBT, Albert Ellis, who considered that it is best for REBT therapists to help clients with their problems straightaway, which, he argued, most clients seem to want.

From a working alliance perspective, if your REBT therapist does not have a preference concerning which approach to take with you, they will make each approach explicit to you and invite you to select the approach that you think will be most helpful to you.

Also, from a collaborative perspective, if your therapist does have a preference concerning which approach to begin with, it is important that they make this clear to you and get your agreement.

Stage 3: Focusing on One Problem at a Time and the Importance of Being Specific

Whether your therapist adopts a formulation-based approach or a problem-based approach to REBT, when you do begin to tackle your problems it is likely to be one at a time and, as you do so, it is also likely that your therapist will ask you to identify a specific example of the nominated problem. The reason for this specificity is that, in general, it provides you both with more valuable information than if you discuss your problems in general terms. You might wish to select a typical example of your nominated problem, a recent example, a vivid example or one that may occur in the near future. The important thing about the selected example is that it helps you and your therapist understand the factors that are at play in your problem. In discussing this specific example of your problem, your therapist may help you to do some or all of the following:

- Describe the situation in which the problem occurred and what you found most difficult about the situation.
- Identify what emotion(s) you felt in the situation.
- Identify how you acted in the situation or how you felt like acting.
- Identify what you did to try to cope with the problem.

In addition, your therapist will help you to set goals with respect to the problem which will help you to know what you are aiming for in similar problematic situations.

Stage 4: Examining Your Rigid/Extreme Attitudes and Develop Flexible/Non-Extreme Alternatives to These Attitudes and Associated Behaviour and Thinking

In REBT, rigid and extreme attitudes are seen to be at the core of your emotional problems. Your therapist will help you to understand the role that such rigid and extreme attitudes have on your problems. They will help you to identify and examine these attitudes and adopt and develop flexible and non-extreme attitude alternatives. As you do this, change will begin to occur.

Your therapist will also encourage you to consider the role that your behaviour and associated thinking play in your problems and will help you to develop more constructive ways of acting and more realistic ways of thinking, as appropriate. When your attitudes are flexible and non-extreme, your behaviour is constructive, your associated thinking is realistic, and you marry the three consistently in dealing with what for you are adversities, then you will experience the therapeutic power of REBT.

Stage 5: Applying What You Learn

What you learn within therapy sessions about the factors that account for the presence of your problems and how you unwittingly maintain them is, of course, a central plank of REBT, for without this you would continue to experience these problems, particularly if they are long-standing. However, unless you apply what you learn from these sessions to your everyday life, then it is unlikely that you will derive any lasting benefit from REBT. This is such an important topic that I have devoted an entire chapter to it (see Chapter 6).

Stage 6: Generalizing Your Gains to Other Problems

Once you have made progress in dealing with your target problems, your therapist will help you to generalize what you have learned to other problems that you would like help with.

Fiona learned in therapy that her anxiety about meeting new people was based on her rigid and extreme attitude (e.g. 'I must not be rejected, and if I am, that would be awful'). To deal with her anxiety, she avoided meeting new people. Her therapist helped Fiona to develop a flexible and non-extreme towards rejection (e.g., 'I don't want to be rejected, but it doesn't have to be the way I want. If I am rejected, that would be bad, but definitely not awful') and then to approach new people while practising this flexible/non-extreme attitude. She did this and as she met new people she experienced a significant decrease in her anxiety. As such, her therapist helped her to apply her learning to her other anxieties, e.g. anxiety about public speaking and taking examinations. She was also encouraged to see that flexible and non-awfulizing thinking would also help her with her jealousy problem, although she had to learn some new skills in dealing with this latter problem.

Stage 7: Maintaining Your Gains

It is tempting to think that once you have made significant progress in dealing with your problems, then therapy is over. However, given the fact that we humans seem to have a talent for lapsing (defined as making slips and returning briefly to the problem) and relapsing (defined as going back to square one), if you do not deal adequately with these slips, then it is likely that you will relapse (see Chapter 8 for more information on this point). It is important, therefore, for you to recognize that you need to make a commitment to work consistently to maintain the benefits that you made in therapy. Also, the more you practise what you have learned in therapy in a deliberate fashion, the more likely it is that these learnings will eventually become second nature to you.

Stage 8: Becoming Your Own REBT Therapist

There is an old adage which states: 'Give a person a fish and you feed them for a day. Teach a person to fish and you feed that person for a lifetime.' If we adapt this to REBT we have: 'If your therapist helps you to solve a problem with REBT, then they will have helped you with that problem. If they teach you how to become your own REBT therapist, then they will have equipped you for life.' Thus, if it is feasible and you are interested, then the final stage of the REBT process involves you learning to be your own REBT therapist. I will discuss this issue in Chapter 8.

At all stages of the change process, you will experience obstacles to change, and these need to be identified and addressed if you are going to get the most out of REBT. I will deal with the most common obstacles to change in Chapter 7. Meanwhile, in the next chapter I will deal with a most important topic: how you can get the most out of REBT in your everyday life by applying what you learn in therapy sessions.

Chapter 6

Apply What You Learn

One of the most robust findings in the scientific literature on REBT and CBT is that people who put into practice between sessions what they learn within sessions get more out of REBT than people who don't do this between-session practice. It follows from this that if you want to get the most out of REBT, then you need to apply what you learn from therapy in your everyday life.

In my view, you need to realize fully that much of what you can achieve from REBT is within your hands and that making a commitment to undertake regular practice of whatever skills you have learned in your therapy sessions is very important if you are going to derive the greatest benefit from REBT.

Let me give you an example of such a commitment from my own life because I think that it details a number of points that are relevant to the importance of undertaking a similar commitment in REBT.

A number of years ago I was diagnosed with a disintegrating disc in my back and later with a torn cartilage in my right knee. I was told that while these two conditions might be helped with surgery, I could manage both myself by doing a number of relevant strengthening exercises. Practising these exercises takes me about 25 minutes every day. I decided from the outset that I would make a commitment to do such practice six days a week.

DOI: 10.4324/9781003493198-7

I do so in the morning before I go for my jog-walk. My decision was underpinned by the following principles:

1. I did not want to subject myself to surgery with its attendant risks and uncertain outcome.
2. I wanted to take responsibility for my own recovery rather than handing over such responsibility to other people.
3. I determined that I would do these exercises whether I wanted to do them or not. I realized that I didn't have to be or feel motivated to do the exercises. I just needed to do them. My behaviour was based on the following flexible/non-extreme attitude: 'It would be nice if I feel motivated to do these exercises but I don't need such motivation. I can and will do them even if I don't feel motivated.'
4. I learned to discriminate between good reasons for not doing the exercises (e.g. 'I am not going to do the exercises because I am ill') and rationalizations for not doing them (e.g. 'I will do the exercises tonight when I have more time to concentrate on them') and I resolved to respond to the latter and then take constructive action (i.e. by doing the exercises).
5. I created favourable environmental conditions that would help me to do the exercises rather than hinder me from doing them. Thus, I set my alarm to help me to get up on time. I make sure that the room where I do the exercises is suitably heated and that the relevant equipment is to hand.

The five principles that I outlined above are very relevant to the issue of you applying what you learn in REBT sessions to your everyday life outside these sessions. Thus:

1. The more you keep in mind the purpose of applying what you learn, the more you will do so. Keep a written reminder

of your goals to hand so you can see the purpose of putting into practice what you have learned in therapy.

2. The more you take responsibility for putting into practice what you learn in therapy, the more you will do this practice.

3. If you resolve to put into practice what you learn in therapy whether preferable conditions exist (e.g. having a feeling that you want to apply what you learn and having a sense of motivation for doing so) or not, then you are much more likely to do such practice than if you insist on the presence of such conditions.

4. The more you monitor your thoughts relating to the possibility of you not putting what you have learned in REBT sessions into practice in your everyday life and the more you learn to stand back and examine such thoughts, the more you will be able to discriminate between proper reasons for not taking action and rationalizations for not doing so. Once you become adept at making such discriminations, you will be able to respond productively to your rationalizations and thus you will probably choose not to act on their content.

5. The more you structure your environment to help you take productive action, the more you will be able to do so. Structuring your environment depends, in part, on your understanding of how to get the best out of yourself with respect to putting your REBT-derived learning into practice. Thus, I am more likely to write when I am in an environment where there is non-intrusive noise and hustle and bustle around me (e.g. while the TV is on or in a coffee bar) than when I am in a silent environment. Consequently, I write while the TV is on or I seek out coffee bars in which to write. Think about the importance of structuring your environment when planning to put into practice what you have learned from your REBT sessions and choose an environment, if possible, that will help you maximize the chances that you will do this practice.

Homework Tasks

REBT therapists often refer to activities that clients undertake to put into practice what they have learned in therapy sessions as 'homework tasks'. Some people, however, do not like the term 'homework' given the negative connotations that it has for them with respect to their school experiences, for example. If this is the case for you, inform your therapist and together choose a term that is more acceptable to you.

In this section, I will deal with two main issues: (i) negotiating homework tasks and (ii) reviewing homework tasks.

Negotiating Homework Tasks

With respect to negotiating homework tasks with you, you can expect your therapist to do the following:

Negotiate a homework task with you. Your therapist will not tell you what to do between therapy sessions. Rather, they will negotiate a suitable homework task with you.

Help ensure that the homework task is a relevant one. Such a task should follow logically from what you have discussed in the therapy session. It may involve you reading something, identifying attitudes, examining such attitudes, imagining acting differently or actually doing so. The type of homework task should also be relevant to the stage reached by the two of you on the problem or issue you are working on together.

Ensure that you understand the nature of the negotiated task and its therapeutic purpose. If you don't understand what you have agreed to do or why you have agreed to do it, it is important that you speak up and say so.

Work with you to select a homework task that is 'challenging, but not overwhelming' for you. Thus, the task should not be too easy for you (and thus of very limited therapeutic power) or too difficult for you (in which case you will not do it).

Introduce and explain the 'no lose' concept of homework tasks to you. Your therapist will explain that if you do the task, then that is good because it is likely that you have benefitted from doing so, and if you don't do the task, good can come out of that too, since this will help you to understand more about both the nature of your problem and the obstacle(s) to making progress. I will discuss this latter issue in Chapter 7.

Ensure that you have the necessary skills to carry out the homework task and believe you can do it. If you lack the skills to carry out a homework task, then no amount of determination will make up for this lack. If you do lack certain skills that are important for you to acquire before you do the task, then your therapist will help you to acquire them. If, on the other hand, your therapist thinks you have such skills in your repertoire and you don't, then it is important that you speak up and tell them.

Allow sufficient time in the session to negotiate the homework task properly with you. Novice REBT therapists know that they 'should' negotiate homework tasks with their clients, but often lose track of time in therapy and realize, often very late, that the therapy session is ending and they have not helped their clients set homework.

Consequently, they panic and often end up by unilaterally 'giving' their clients homework tasks rather than taking their time to negotiate such tasks properly with their clients. If your therapist is experienced, then they will manage the session sufficiently to enable them to spend time on negotiating a suitable homework task with you. If not – and don't forget your therapist is human – remind them about the topic of homework if it looks as if they may have forgotten.

Elicit a firm commitment from you that you will carry out the homework task. It is one thing for you to agree to carry out a homework task, it is another thing to commit yourself to doing so. Thus, you can expect your REBT therapist to ask you for a firm commitment to do the task that you have both negotiated and to explore any reluctance that you have to do so.

Help you specify when, where and how often you will carry out the homework task. The more specific you can be concerning when, where and how often you will carry out the negotiated homework task, the more likely it is that you will do so. Thus, you can expect your therapist to ask you to give them such specific undertakings. Otherwise, you may be tempted to delay carrying out the task, perhaps leaving it till the last minute. If this happens, it will mean, in all probability, that you won't get the most out of doing the agreed task.

Encourage you to make a written note of the homework task and its relevant details and to refer to it when appropriate. When clients do not carry out their homework tasks, one of the main reasons they give is that they forgot what the homework was and that they hadn't made a written note of the task. Thus, you can expect your therapist to ask you to make a written note of the agreed task and to suggest that you refer to this written note periodically so that you do not forget what it was when you come to do it.

Elicit from you the potential obstacles to homework completion and help you deal in advance with any such obstacles. In the next chapter, I will discuss the more general issue of why you may not be making as much progress in REBT as you may reasonably expect. One of the main reasons for lack of progress is failure to complete homework tasks. Thus, you can expect your therapist to explore with you, in advance, possible obstacles to homework completion and how these might be dealt with. If you have continued difficulty in carrying out such tasks, I suggest that you fill out the appropriate form in Appendix 3 and discuss your responses with your therapist.

Help you to rehearse the homework task in the session, if practicable. If doing so is practicable and there is sufficient time, then your therapist may suggest that you rehearse your agreed homework task in the therapy session. The reason for this is twofold. First, it gives you experience of doing the task in controlled conditions so you can get a sense of what doing it in the outside world might be like. Second, it may help you and your therapist to identify and problem-solve an obstacle to carrying out the task not already identified.

Reviewing Homework Tasks

Unless you review your homework tasks with your therapist in subsequent sessions, it is unlikely that you will consider them to have the level of importance that they actually have in REBT. Again, it is worthwhile keeping in mind that one of the most robust research findings in REBT and CBT is that people who routinely carry out homework tasks get a lot more out of the process than those who do not. With this in mind, with respect to reviewing homework tasks with you, you can expect your therapist to do the following:

Check with you whether or not you did the homework task. Unless your therapist checks with you concerning whether or not you did the task and what your experiences of doing so were, then they will be implicitly communicating to you that doing such tasks are not important in REBT when, in reality, they are. Such a review is usually done at the beginning of the next session so that you can usefully prepare what you are going to say about doing (or not doing) the task in advance of the session, as I discussed in Chapter 4.

Determine the reasons why you did not do the task as agreed, if this was the case, and address with you any obstacles. If you did not do the homework task, then you may expect your therapist to explore with you the reasons for this. You might usefully prepare for this discussion by completing the form to be found in Appendix 3 and bringing your responses to therapy. Ideally, your therapist's stance here should be to be genuinely interested in identifying any obstacles to homework completion with a view to helping you to address these obstacles rather than reprimanding you for not doing the task. If the latter is the case, speak up if you can and tell your therapist that their stance is not helpful to you. I will discuss the issue of you speaking up and giving your therapist feedback in greater detail in Chapter 7.

Check whether you made any modification(s) to the task and, if so, determine the reasons for the modification(s). You may have done your homework task, and you may have thought you had done so successfully, but you may have changed the task to make it easier for you to carry it out. In doing so, you may have reduced the therapeutic power of the task. Given this, you may expect your therapist to enquire in some detail about what you actually did to determine whether or not this was the case. If it was, your therapist will help you to discover what led you to make the modification and to deal with this factor if it helps you unwittingly to maintain your problem. It is important that your therapist acknowledges what you achieved by doing the task as well as pointing out to you the problems raised by the modification you made to it.

Bernice agreed to deal with her anxiety about going shopping and losing control in supermarkets by practising her newly developed flexible/non-extreme attitude towards not feeling in control and doing so on her own in a supermarket without access to support from others. She reported that she did this and that the prospect of losing control seemed more manageable. However, on closer questioning, Bernice admitted that during the task she had phoned her daughter for support and, even though she did not speak to her daughter, she gained support from knowing that her daughter was there on the open phone line should she need her.

Her therapist acknowledged the stride forward that Bernice had made by going to the supermarket on her own, but discussed with her that she only thought that she could do so if she had direct contact with her daughter. This led to an exploration of Bernice's thoughts about doing the task without such support and she negotiated a new task where she went to the supermarket without her mobile phone based on the work she and her therapist did on the thoughts she had about the original task.

Review what you learned from doing the task. Doing the task as agreed is important, of course, but what you learned from doing so is, in some ways, more important. So, expect your therapist to ask you what you learned from doing the task. Sometimes what you learned may not be that helpful to you. Thus, you may learn from giving a public speech as a homework task that nobody laughed at you and that nobody will laugh when you give a speech. While it is good for you to learn that nobody laughed when you predicted that everybody would, it is unreasonable to jump to the conclusion that nobody will laugh in future. Here, your therapist might suggest that it would be helpful to prepare for being laughed at even though this event may be unlikely.

Deal with homework 'failure'. You may have done the task and derived no benefit from it and thus you may consider the homework to have been a failure. As discussed earlier in this section, there are times when your therapist will carefully examine what you did, what happened and your thinking about the experience, and exploring homework 'failure' is one of those times. Remember what I said earlier in this

chapter about the 'no lose' concept of homework completion. If your homework was a 'failure', then that is bad, but
the good thing to come out of it is understanding the reasons
for the failure and using what you and your therapist discover in this process to help yourself more effectively in the
future.

Capitalize on your success. While I have concentrated on
some of the difficulties that you might experience in the area
of homework tasks in REBT, I want to stress that very often
clients do their tasks as agreed and gain a lot from doing so.
When this happens, you can expect that your therapist will
help you to capitalize on your success and encourage you
to use your derived learning to further your progress on the
problems that you are focusing on and perhaps to apply this
learning to your other problems as well.

Applying what you learn from therapy sessions to your
everyday life is the heart of REBT, in my view. However, as we
have seen, REBT does not always go smoothly, and in the next
chapter, I will focus on the issues that emerge when you don't
make the expected progress from your therapy.

Chapter 7

Understand and Deal with Lack of Progress

Sometimes in therapy people do not make the progress that they can be expected to have made and it is important that you realize that this may happen with you. If it does occur, you should ideally be prepared to join your therapist in looking for reasons for such lack of progress and in dealing with these obstacles to change accordingly. In this chapter, I will consider some of the common reasons for lack of progress and suggest ways in which you can best deal with them.[1] I will use the following structure in this chapter:

- Lack of progress due to problems in the working alliance.
- Lack of progress due to client factors.
- Lack of progress due to therapist factors.

I will discuss the most common obstacles to progress that occur in each of the above categories before discussing the more general issue of how you and your therapist can address such obstacles.

Lack of Progress due to Problems in the Working Alliance

Having a good working alliance with your therapist is what sustains therapy over the course, and thus if you are not making progress, it is important that you and your therapist investigate the possibility that there is a problem in the alliance that needs addressing.

DOI: 10.4324/9781003493198-8

The Therapeutic Bond Between You and Your Therapist Is Not Good

The bonding aspect of the working alliance concerns the feeling tone that exists in the relationship between you and your therapist. Thus, if you don't have good feelings for one another, this may have a negative effect on your progress. My view is that while you can still make progress in therapy if you and your therapist don't like one another, it is more difficult to do so if there is no mutual respect or if you do not have confidence in your therapist's expertise.

The Therapeutic Bond Between You and Your Therapist Is Too Good

You may think it strange that getting on too well might be a reason why you may not be making progress in REBT, but it certainly can happen. You and your therapist may enjoy each other's company so much that you may drift away from the primary objective concerning why you are seeking therapy – to address your emotional problems.

I introduced the following points in Chapter 3 when I was talking about the therapeutic agreements that you need to make with your therapist in REBT, but since disagreements on these points may explain lack of progress, I will discuss them briefly here (see also Chapter 3). Please note that while the disagreements that I discuss below may be clear and explicitly stated, they are more often implicit and therefore not stated.

You and Your Therapist Disagree on the Nature of Your Problem(s)

If you consider that you have a problem with guilt, for example, while your therapist considers that your problem is one of shame, you may end up by talking at cross purposes, and since these two emotions are underpinned by different attitudes and associated with different behaviours, this may result in you focusing on the wrong factors and may result in lack of progress.

You and Your Therapist Disagree about the Goals of Therapy

You and your therapist may agree on the nature of your problem but may disagree concerning the goals of therapy with respect to this problem. Thus, you both may agree that you have a problem with unhealthy suppressed anger, for example, but while you think that the goal of therapy should be to help you to get your anger out of your system, your therapist may think that the goal should be to help you to express yourself with respectful annoyance. If this is the case, you will be going in one direction while your therapist will be going in another, which again may result in lack of progress.

You and Your Therapist Have Disagreements about the Focus of Therapy

While nothing is ruled out when it comes to you discussing your problems, as I pointed out in Chapter 1, the focus of REBT is largely on the present and the future, and when the past is discussed it is done so in a way that facilitates understanding of these two foci. Thus, if you want to discuss your past experiences extensively without regard to the present and the future, then you may not make progress if your therapist does not join you in a comprehensive examination of your past. REBT theory would also hypothesize that you may not make much progress even if your therapist does join you in this exploration, since while you are going over the past with them, you are still being influenced by the attitude and behavioural factors that underpin your problems both in the present and going forward into the future.

You and Your Therapist Disagree about Your Respective Roles

As discussed in Chapter 3, REBT involves you and your therapist both adopting an active and collaborative role in therapy, and when this does not happen for any reason, you may not make as much therapeutic progress as when it does. While the most common occurrence on this issue concerns the client not assuming an active role, it may also happen that a therapist may not be active in the process or may fail to be sufficiently collaborative with the client.

You and Your Therapist Disagree about Therapeutic Tasks or Experience Other Problems about These Tasks

Therapeutic tasks are activities that you and your therapist engage in with the purpose of helping you to achieve your therapeutic goals. If you both do not agree that undertaking these tasks is helpful, then this may compromise your progress. Even if you do agree on this point, things may go wrong, as shown in the following vignette.

Gerald was seeking help from an REBT therapist for depression and readily agreed with the REBT-based conceptualization of his problems. His therapist taught him to use a form that was designed to help people identify and respond to rigid and extreme attitudes that underpin depression, and Gerald could see the sense of doing this. However, Gerald had very poor spelling, about which he was ashamed, and this resulted in his not completing the forms as requested by his therapist. His sense of shame prevented him from bringing up this obstacle with his therapist.

Lack of Progress due to Client Factors

When I say that you may be largely responsible for your lack of progress, it is not to blame you but to help you to address such obstacles fair and square. With that in mind, let's look at some common client obstacles to change.

You Believe That Change Is Not Possible

If you think that change is not possible, you will not engage fully with the REBT process. Consequently, you will not get as much out of the process as you would do if you do thought that you could change.

You Opt for Short-Term 'Solutions' to Your Problem(s)

We, as human beings, generally seek to make ourselves comfortable whenever we experience discomfort, and this is not a problem for us as long as there is no good reason for experiencing such discomfort. Since achieving your therapeutic goals generally involves discomfort, then unless you are prepared to experience such discomfort your progress will be very limited. Signs that you are opting for the short-term solution of getting rid of the discomfort associated with your problem rather than being prepared to experience discomfort in the short term while facing your problem and dealing with it are many but include: denying that you have a problem, overcompensating for your problem and using safety-seeking behaviours to avoid experiencing your problem.

Luke was anxious about meeting new people, especially in social settings. In order to deal with this problem, Luke would (i) avoid such occasions, or, if he could not do so, he would (ii) pretend that he had lost his voice so he did not have to speak to people. He would also (iii) consume quite a lot of alcohol to 'take the edge off' his anxiety, as he put it. In REBT, his therapist helped him to see that while these three behaviours kept his anxiety at bay in the short term, they did not help him deal with his anxiety problem in the longer term. Luke learned more adaptive ways of dealing with his anxiety by developing a set of flexible/non-extreme attitudes and resolved to put this learning into practice rather than use the three short-term 'solutions'. However, Luke did not make as much progress as possible because it transpired that he managed to get one of his friends invitations to these social events and spent time with that person rather than talking to people whom he did not know while practising the REBT skills that he learned in his therapy sessions and agreed to practise for homework.

You Have Doubts, Reservations and Objections to Aspects of Your Therapy That You Do Not Disclose

REBT is based on a particular way of making sense of your problems, of explaining how you may have unwittingly maintained these problems and of determining what you need to do to address them effectively. In order to get the most out of REBT, you need to collaborate with your therapist in developing these problem-based and therapy-based understandings. When you don't make as much progress as expected, it may be due to one or more doubts, reservations or objections that you have with respect to these understandings that you have not expressed, the existence of which have negatively affected your participation in therapy.

Carol had a problem with chronic guilt and was easily manipulated by others, with the result that she would always put others before herself. She worked closely with her REBT therapist to develop an REBT-based conceptualization of her problems and, together, they worked to devise a way of addressing these problems effectively. However, despite doing all her agreed homework tasks, Carol did not make much progress in therapy. After therapy finished, Carol admitted to her friend that she had several doubts about the treatment plan that she, at least on the surface, was involved in developing with her therapist. She told her friend that she did not tell her therapist her doubts because she did not want to upset her therapist. This was the case even though her therapist had asked her if she had any doubts, reservations or objections to any aspect of therapy.

You Think That Intellectual Insight Is Enough to Help You

In REBT there are two forms of insight, what might be termed 'intellectual insight' and 'emotional insight'. When you have intellectual insight, you understand and agree with the REBT concepts that you are being taught but this insight has not yet impacted on your feelings and behaviour. Emotional insight, on the other hand, does impact on your feelings and behaviour. Thus, you may know that making an important error does not make you a less worthwhile person, but this insight (intellectual) will not impact on your feelings and behaviour until you act on it and keep doing so until you come to believe it. Thus, you may not make much progress in REBT if you believe that intellectual insight is enough to achieve your goals.

You Are Not Prepared to Work for Change

As I have discussed throughout this book, REBT depends on you taking an active role in the therapeutic process both inside and outside the therapy room. So, if you are not prepared to work for change, then you will not make very much progress. Here are some common progress-blocking attitudes that people have in this area:

- 'I shouldn't have to help myself; it is my therapist's job to help me.'
- 'I'm too lazy to help myself.'
- 'I don't have the time to carry out homework tasks.'

If you hold these or similar attitudes, you need to discuss them with your therapist.

You Are Intolerant of the Discomfort and Unfamiliarity Associated with Change

While you can achieve a lot from REBT, you will not do so unless (i) you are prepared for the discomfort of facing up to and discussing painful issues and (ii) you are prepared to tolerate the unfamiliarity that you will experience during the process of change. As I often say: 'If it isn't strange, it isn't change.' So if you are intolerant of such discomfort and feelings of unnaturalness, then you will not make much progress in REBT, and to remedy this, you need to discuss this with your therapist.

Lack of Progress due to Therapist Factors

So far, I have discussed possible reasons why you have not made much progress in REBT that are due to problems in the working alliance that you have with your therapist or due to factors within you as a client. However, your therapist may be largely responsible for your lack of progress, and I will briefly discuss some of these therapist factors in this section.

Your Therapist Lacks Important General Therapeutic Skills

One of the most common therapist factors that impedes client progress is that the therapist lacks general therapeutic skills. When a therapist lacks general therapeutic skills:

- They fail to listen to you or empathize with you.
- They consistently put words into your mouth.
- They interact with you in a way that reinforces your problems (e.g. they are too active, and this reinforces your problematic passivity).
- They have unreasonably high or unreasonably low expectations of you, which results in them either pushing you too much or too little.
- They are too forceful in making points and fail to elicit or take into account your views.
- They misjudge what stage of change you are in and work with you in the wrong stage of change (e.g. they assume that you are ready to change something when you are, in fact, ambivalent about doing so).

Your Therapist Lacks REBT-Specific Skills

One of the other most common therapist factors that impedes client progress is that the therapist lacks REBT-specific skills. This is why it is important that you check the credentials of your REBT therapist, as there are many therapists who say that they practise REBT when they are not fully qualified to do so. However, consulting a qualified REBT therapist, while important, is no guarantee that the therapist will not lack core REBT-specific skills. When a therapist lacks such skills:

- They fail to understand accurately your problems in REBT terms.

- They fail to explain clearly their understanding of your problems even if their understanding is accurate.
- They fail to suggest an REBT approach that, if you both use it properly, will help you deal effectively with your problems.
- They suggest an effective REBT approach to your problems but implement this poorly.
- They are poor in negotiating and reviewing suitable homework tasks.
- They do not identify and address effectively reasons why you may not be making expected progress in REBT.

Your Therapist Has Personal Issues/Problems That Interfere with Them Helping You

It is important for you to recognize that your therapist is human and is not immune from the problems and issues that all human beings are capable of experiencing. Having said that, it is realistic for you to expect that whatever problems your therapist may have will not intrude on your therapy. Sadly, this is not always the case, and here are some examples where the therapist's issues/problems do interfere with therapy and may help to explain your lack of progress:

- Your therapist has the same problem as you and has not been able to help themself with that problem, with the result that they fail to offer you credible help.
- Your therapist believes that they need your approval, with the result that they fail to confront you appropriately.
- Your therapist believes that their worth depends on your progress, with the result that they may get angry or defensive if you don't make the progress that they expect.
- Your therapist has a problem with impatience and seems to get impatient or irritable if you fail to understand something or when therapy does not go smoothly.

- Your therapist disturbs themself about your problems, with the result that they cannot gain the professional distance they need to help you effectively.

Dealing with Lack of Progress

When you are not making as much progress as you might reasonably expect for one or more of the reasons discussed above (or for other reasons), it is important that you and your therapist address this issue. If you do not do so, it is unlikely that you will be able, on your own, to overcome these obstacles to progress.

Most people would say, rightly in my view, that it is mainly your therapist's responsibility to initiate a discussion concerning these reasons, even if you have brought up the issue of lack of progress in the first place. However, you also have a responsibility to speak up, since your therapist will not be able to read your mind and deal with matters without your active participation in this process. I will discuss both your and your therapist's responsibility for dealing with lack of progress in the rest of this chapter.

Your Therapist's Responsibility for Dealing with Lack of Progress

If your therapist thinks that you are not making progress as expected, then it is important that they bring this to your attention and initiate a discussion about this. Your therapist should preferably also initiate such a discussion when you have brought up the issue of lack of progress. When initiating such a discussion, this will go better if your therapist has already established what is known as a 'meta-therapy dialogue' with you. This is a technical term which refers to a process where you and your therapist stand back, as it were, and reflect on issues pertaining to therapy. If your therapist has already set up such a dialogue with you, then the subsequent discussion about lack of progress should go more smoothly than if such a dialogue has not yet been established.

Once the discussion about lack of progress has been initiated, there are two major things that your therapist needs to do to increase the chances that this discussion will be fruitful.

Your Therapist Needs to Adopt a Flexible and Negotiable Stance in the Discussion

When your therapist adopts such a flexible stance, then you will say things like:

- 'My therapist and I are good at finding a solution if we disagree.'
- 'I do not feel that I have to pretend to agree with my therapist's goals for our therapy so that the sessions run smoothly.'
- 'I feel like I have a say regarding what we do in therapy.'
- 'My therapist is flexible and takes my wants or needs into consideration.'
- 'I do not feel that my therapist tells me what to do and has regard for my wants or needs.'
- 'My therapist is flexible in their ideas regarding what we do in therapy.'

As you can see from the above statements, when your therapist establishes a flexible and negotiable stance, this will help both of you to reflect on the reasons for your lack of expected progress as a client. Compare this with what you are likely to say if your therapist is rigid and not open to negotiation about possible reasons for your lack of progress.

- 'I feel that my therapist tells me what to do, without much regard for my wants or needs.'
- 'My therapist is inflexible and does not take my wants or needs into consideration.'

- 'My therapist is rigid in their ideas regarding what we do in therapy.'
- 'I feel like I do not have a say regarding what we do in therapy.'
- 'I pretend to agree with my therapist's goals for our therapy so the session runs smoothly.'
- 'My therapist and I are not good at finding a solution if we disagree about what we should be working on in therapy.'

Indeed, if your therapist routinely displays such closed-mindedness, this may be a prime reason for your lack of progress. Most therapists at times show a closed-minded attitude, but if yours does so routinely, then you may need to consult a different REBT therapist!

Your Therapist Needs to Demonstrate That They Are Comfortable Dealing with Disagreement and with Any Negative Feelings That You Might Express

When you therapist demonstrates such comfort, then you will say things like:

- 'I feel that I can disagree with my therapist without harming our relationship.'
- 'My therapist encourages me to express any concerns I have with our progress.'
- 'I am comfortable expressing disappointment in my therapist when it arises.'
- 'My therapist encourages me to express any anger I feel towards them.'
- 'My therapist is able to admit when they are wrong about something we disagree on.'
- 'I am comfortable expressing frustration with my therapist when it arises.'

As you can see from these statements, if your therapist can comfortably hear and, indeed, invite your negativity about

aspects of the therapy and the way in which they are working with you, you are likely to feel able, in turn, to be honest
about your negative feelings about your lack of progress and the
things that may be hindering such progress. You will also feel
free to say what you don't like about the therapy.

Compare this with what you are likely to say if your therapist is uncomfortable dealing with disagreement and with your
negative feelings about them or your therapy.

- 'I don't feel that I can disagree with my therapist without
  harming our relationship.'
- 'My therapist does not encourage me to express any concerns
  I have with our progress.'
- 'I am not comfortable expressing disappointment in my ther-
  apist when it arises.'
- 'My therapist does not encourage me to express any anger
  I feel towards them.'
- 'My therapist is unable to admit when they are wrong about
  something we disagree on.'
- 'I am not comfortable expressing frustration with my ther-
  apist when it arises.'

The chances are that you will be reluctant to be honest about
your thoughts and feelings about why you may not be progress-
ing in therapy. Most therapists at times show discomfort about
disagreement and about hearing something negative about
therapy, but again, if yours does so routinely, a change of REBT
therapist may be in order!

Your Therapist Needs to Give You Honest Feedback about How Therapy Is Proceeding and What Factors Might Explain Your Lack of Progress

As well as being able to take bad news as demonstrated above,
your therapist also needs to be able to give bad news in offer-
ing their opinion about why you may not be making expected

progress. A good therapist has the ability to be honest without discouraging you in the process. Thus, if your therapist considers that a major reason for your lack of progress is your failure to apply yourself in a consistent way to carrying out homework tasks, then they should say so, but in a way that shows that you could apply yourself and, as importantly, in a way that engages you in an honest exploration of why you may not be applying yourself as consistently as you might. I should add that it is particularly important for your therapist to be honest if you have unreasonable expectations about change and you are, in fact, making as much progress as you might be expected to be making. Encouraging you to develop more realistic expectations about progress may help you to re-invest in the process of REBT and make advances in a slower, but perhaps more sustained manner.

If your therapist does not give you genuine feedback, they may be depriving you of the opportunity to address some uncomfortable truths which, if addressed, may well help you to make more progress in therapy.

Your Responsibility for Dealing with Lack of Progress

Having outlined what responsibility your therapist has in dealing with your lack of progress, let me be clear and state that you also have responsibility here. My view is that your responsibility is to speak up and be honest. Yes, as we have seen, your therapist can facilitate or hinder you in this regard, but no matter how facilitative your therapist is, you still have a choice whether or not to speak up and be honest. You may well be apprehensive about being assertive in this regard for fear of hurting your therapist's feelings, for example, but if you don't take the risk, particularly when your therapist has demonstrated their flexibility and comfort in dealing with difficult issues, then remember this: your therapist can't help you with something about which they do not know.

However, if you don't feel able to speak up and be honest about something that may be hindering your progress in therapy, then you can talk about your difficulty about doing so. In this, your therapist can help in two ways. First, they can help you overcome your fear of speaking up, and then when you have spoken up, they can help you with whatever you have spoken up about.

Violet was seeking help for a chronic problem with pro-crastination. She was making good progress with this until her therapist put forward the hypothesis that a com-ponent of her problem was due to autonomy issues. She privately disagreed with this hypothesis but told her ther-apist that she agreed. It was when she stopped making progress that her therapist encouraged a discussion about possible reasons for this. During this discussion, Violet told her therapist that she found it difficult to be honest with him. He helped her to investigate this with him and then encouraged her to tell him that she thought he was wrong about his autonomy hypothesis. He demonstrated comfort with this feedback, and with therapy properly recalibrated, she began to make progress again.

By identifying and addressing the reasons for your lack of progress, you should be able to make the progress you were expecting and eventually achieve your goals. When this happens, it may be time to end therapy. However, you also have the possibility, if practicable, of learning how to be your own therapist, and I will discuss this issue in the following chapter.

Note

1 In this chapter, when I discuss lack of progress, I refer to instances when you are not making as much progress as you might reasonably be expected to be making. You may, of course, have unreasonable expectations of progress with respect to your problems and are, in fact, making expected progress. This is something that your therapist will discuss with you, as I will make clear later in the chapter.

Chapter 8

Become Your Own REBT Therapist

One of the major goals that your REBT therapist is likely to have is to help you to become your own REBT therapist. This means that you will be helped to develop a number of skills which you will be encouraged to use increasingly for yourself over the course of therapy with the aim of using them for yourself when formal therapy has ended.

While this is a major aim of REBT, it is important to note that as a client you may or may not be interested in learning to use REBT-based self-help skills for yourself after therapy has ended, or if you are, you may be interested in doing this informally in your own way and may not wish to learn these skills in a more structured, formal way. The important point, and one that I have stressed throughout this book, is that effective REBT therapists are prepared to tailor their approaches according to their clients' idiosyncratic situations and preferences. Having said that, in this final chapter, I am going to discuss what you can expect from REBT if you are interested to learn how to become your own REBT therapist. In doing so, I will not discuss specific skills that may or may not be relevant to you; rather, I will focus on categories of skills that are likely to have broader relevance.

Learning Assessment Skills

When you are working towards becoming your own REBT therapist, it is important that you learn how to identify the

DOI: 10.4324/9781003493198-9

important factors that comprise your reactions to situations that are problematic for you. As part of this process, your therapist may suggest that you use a printed form on which there will be a number of headings and spaces under those headings for you to write down your responses. There are a number of such forms and the one suggested by your therapist and the one you suggest may be dictated by their preferences as a therapist and/ or the nature of your problem(s) for which you are seeking help.

Assessment forms are usually designed to help you to assess specific information. They may or may not include information detailing how to complete them. Once you have filled out such a form on a number of occasions, you will be able to see more general patterns emerge that will help you to anticipate how you may respond so that you can help yourself early on in a problem episode or even in advance of a likely episode. I will discuss this in greater detail later in this chapter.

Filling in such forms and thus learning to assess your problems involves you being able to do the following:

- Identify the kind of situations you find difficult (e.g. speaking in public).
- Identify what you find particularly disturbing about these situations (e.g. your mind going blank). This is your adversity at A.
- Identify the main troublesome emotions at C that you experience in these situations and the major physiological expressions of these feelings, if relevant.
- Identify the behaviours that you carry out to avoid these situations (or what you find troublesome about them) and the behaviours that you carry out when you are in these situations which may make your problems worse. Here, you will also be helped to assess what happens in response to your behaviours.
- Identify how you 'feel like' acting in these situations but do not convert into overt behaviour.

- Identify your distorted thinking that accompanies your troublesome emotions.
- Identify your rigid and extreme attitudes towards the adversity that account for your troublesome emotions and unconstructive behaviour. These are your *B*asic attitudes.

Initially, it is likely that you will be shown how to use the assessment form in a therapy session using a recent problem episode. Here, your therapist will take the lead and guide you towards identifying the relevant information by asking you focused questions. They will then probably ask you to complete a new assessment form before the next therapy session on another specific problem episode and will go over your responses at the beginning of that session. They will then give you feedback to help you to use the form more accurately. This process will continue to the point where you can use the form on your own.

After you have become proficient at using the form, you will find that you may be able to carry out an assessment in your head by referring to its categories either before you encounter a troublesome situation or even while you are in the midst of one. If you need help to do this, ask your therapist, if they do not offer such help themself.

Learning How to Examine Your Attitudes

Here, your therapist will help you to learn how to examine the rigid and extreme attitudes that underpin your problems and the flexible and non-extreme alternative attitudes. In my view, the best way you can learn these skills of attitude examination is in a structured way.

Here is one way of doing this:

- Your therapist will invite you to take your rigid attitude and the flexible attitude alternative.[1]

- Your therapist will encourage you to consider these attitudes together and ask you the following questions.

  ○ Which attitude is true and which is false and why?
  ○ Which attitude is logical and which is illogical and why?
  ○ Which attitude is helpful and which is unhelpful and why?
  ○ Which attitude would you teach your children and why?

- After you have learned to do this on paper, your therapist will encourage you to use this skill in your head, first in imagery and then in actual situations.

While REBT largely focuses on helping clients to develop flexible and non-extreme attitudes, your therapist will also want to teach you other skills either when you get stuck using attitude examination skills or after you have derived benefit from applying such skills.

Learning 'Acceptance-Based' Thinking Skills

Acceptance-based thinking skills are not generally taught by using written forms; rather, they are taught experientially (i.e., by gaining experience in the use of such skills). Here, you may be asked to identify a meaningful metaphor which helps you to digest the idea that you can recognize the existence of something without engaging with it, on the one hand, and without trying to eliminate it, on the other. Your therapist will introduce you to various exercises which will help you to develop these acceptance-based thinking skills and you will be expected to practise these skills in relevant situations. How and at what rate you do this is a matter for negotiation between you and your therapist. Finally, you will be encouraged to practise these skills while pursuing value-based goals.

Learning Behavioural Skills

Another area in which you can learn to be your own REBT therapist involves you acquiring key behavioural skills which will help you to achieve and maintain your goals. Commonly taught behavioural skills in REBT include communication, assertion and study skills.

Communication Skills

Here you learn, among others, how to:

- Listen actively to what others say.
- Convey your understanding of what they are saying.
- State clearly what you want to say.

These skills are particularly important to developing and maintaining good relationships with others.

Assertion Skills

Here, you learn how to state clearly your position on various matters, which serves to help you to maintain healthy boundaries between yourself and others. Assertion skills enable you (i) to convey your negative feelings to others while showing respect for them and, equally important, they also enable you (ii) to convey your positive feelings to them. The skills in the first category are particularly relevant for you if you often do what you don't want to do and therefore get taken advantage of in relationships, and the skills in the second category are more relevant for you if other people complain that you always focus on negative aspects of your relationships to the exclusion of the positive aspects.

Study Skills

Here you learn, among others, how to:

- Organize what you have to do on a course of study.
- Digest information.
- Convey your ideas in writing to enable you to achieve your academic goals.

These are just a sample of behavioural skills that you can learn in REBT if you lack such skills in your behavioural repertoire and the acquisition of such skills is important in helping you to achieve and maintain your therapeutic goals.

The Process of Learning Behavioural Skills

While your REBT therapist will help you to learn and internalize the above-mentioned skills in ways that best suit your learning style, acquiring behavioural skills as part of becoming your own REBT therapist is likely to involve some or all of the following steps:

- Your therapist will help you identify the relevant behavioural skill deficit and encourage you to see how learning this skill will help you to achieve your therapeutic goals and how doing so will stand you in good stead for the future. As part of this process, you will be encouraged to share any doubts, reservations or objections to learning the skill which your therapist will discuss with you in full.
- Your therapist will then outline the skill and break it down into its constituent parts and will model this skill for you if necessary and where practicable.
- You will then try out the skill, first in the therapy session if this can be done, and be encouraged to implement the skill in your own personal style.

- Then, you will be encouraged to practise the skill before the next therapy session.
- You will report back on your experiences of implementing the skill and be given feedback on how to refine it.
- Through this process of skill practice and refinement, based on experience and feedback, you will internalize this skill and be able to use it in the future whenever you need to do so.
- During this process of behavioural skill learning and practice, you may encounter a variety of obstacles along the way. I refer you to Chapter 7, where I devoted an entire chapter to identifying and dealing with obstacles to making progress in REBT. I want to make the point here that you should be prepared to disclose such obstacles to skill learning and internalization to your therapist so that together you may understand and respond effectively to the factors leading to the obstacle.

Learning Emotion Regulation Skills

A recent development in REBT and CBT has been the focus that therapists place on helping clients to regulate their distressed emotions so that they don't feel overwhelmed by them. Some of the skills that I have already discussed form a part of your learning to regulate your emotions. Thus, looking for and responding to the attitudes that underpin your distressed emotions will generally help to abate them, as will externalizing them in some way, as it is often the act of suppressing these emotions that adds to distress. Thus, communicating respectfully how you feel to another person helps in this regard, as does writing your feelings down. In addition, learning to use mindfulness-based skills, where you acknowledge the presence of your distressed emotion and continue to pursue your goals without engaging with the emotion or trying to eliminate it, often serves to reduce the subjective nature of your distress.

In addition to these methods, your therapist may use some or all of the following to teach you how to regulate your own distressing emotions.

Developing Unconditional Self-Acceptance

You might find a negative emotion particularly distressing because you are judging yourself negatively for experiencing the emotion. The presence of shame for having a feeling is a good sign that you are doing this (e.g. regarding yourself as childish and less worthwhile for feeling hurt). Here, your REBT therapist will teach you to accept yourself as an ordinary person experiencing an understandable emotion and help you to see that judging yourself on the basis of an experience is neither valid nor helpful to you.

Learning Self-Validation and Self-Compassion

Self-validation occurs when you are able to reassure yourself that what you feel inside is real, is important and makes sense given the circumstances in which you felt it. Self-compassion extends this in three ways, as noted by the psychologist Dr Kristin Neff: (i) by relating to yourself with kindness, (ii) by encouraging yourself to see that you are not different from others but are a part of common humanity, as we all struggle with distressing feelings at times, and (iii) by encouraging the development of a mindful stance for your feelings (as noted above). Your therapist will help you to take these concepts and to use them in everyday ways and suggest the same process of (i) practice, (ii) feedback and (iii) refinement that I discussed earlier in this chapter.

In my view, it is best if your therapist helps you to accept yourself first before encouraging you to use the skills of self-validation and self-compassion.

Increasing Distress Tolerance

One of the major reasons why you may find your emotions difficult to regulate is that your stance towards them indicates that you find them intolerable. As a result, you may try to get rid of them or away from them as soon as you begin to experience them or you may attempt to avoid situations in which you predict that you might experience them. Some CBT therapists call this 'experiential avoidance', where you literally attempt to avoid experiencing certain emotions. In order to develop a sense of regulation over these emotions, you need to increase your level of tolerance for these emotions. As you do so, you will become less fearful of the emotions and this will help you to deal with the issues that underpin them.

Using Imagery to Deal with Feelings

Approaches to REBT not only focus on thinking that occurs in words; they also focus on thinking that occurs in images. Your therapist can thus help you to use imagery by picturing yourself in troublesome situations and dealing constructively with the feelings that you predict you will experience. Rehearsing such scenarios will help you to become less afraid of your feelings and to face them rather than avoid them.

Using Self-Soothing Skills

In the same way that a mother soothes her baby when the child is upset, you can utilize your five senses to learn to soothe yourself as a means of regulating your distressing emotions.

Learning Relapse Prevention Skills

One very important way in which you can be your own therapist is by learning relapse prevention skills. These involve the following:

- Accepting without liking the reality of lapses or slips (i.e. temporary and non-serious return to your problems).
- Identifying vulnerability factors (i.e. factors both in the environment and inside you that serve as triggers to lapses/slips).
- Developing and rehearsing constructive responses to these vulnerability factors.
- Facing up to these vulnerability factors in a sensible way so that you can practise these constructive responses.
- Accepting yourself if you relapse (i.e. a more serious and enduring return to your problems) and learning from this experience.

Learning to Generalize Your Learning, Becoming Less Prone to Emotional Disturbance in the Future and Pursuing Healthy Self-Development

Whether you have sought help from your REBT therapist for one problem or for several problems, you still have the option to add to your skills as your own therapist once you have achieved what you were seeking from REBT. First, you can generalize your learning; second, you can learn to become less prone to emotional disturbance in the future; and third, you can pursue matters of healthy self-development.

Before I discuss these three issues, I want to make clear that addressing them in therapy is dependent on three points: (i) whether or not you want to learn these skills, (ii) whether or not your therapist conceives working with these issues as being a part of their role and (iii) whether or not the context in which you are seeing your therapist permits such work, given the amount of time that needs to be devoted to it.

As with other matters, you need to discuss such issues with your therapist and come to an agreement on them. However, assuming that both of you want to and are able to focus on such issues and, if relevant, you have the support of the organization in which you are being seen, then the following points should be borne in mind.

Learning to Generalize Your Learning

Once you have achieved your therapeutic goal, or one of them if you have several, then you have the option of generalizing the learning that you derived from achieving your goal(s) to tackling other problems that you may have. You do this by working with your therapist to identify what you learned, to see if this learning is appropriate to your other problems, and determining a plan based on your learning to tackle these problems, if relevant. Answering the following questions may help you in your discussions with your therapist.

- What recurring attitudes, thoughts and images did I identify as being at the core of my problem(s) and how did I respond constructively to them? Are these attitudes, thoughts and images relevant to my other problems and, if so, would responding to them in a similar way also have a constructive impact as I deal with my new problems? If so, how can I best do so?
- What recurring behavioural patterns did I identify as being relevant in understanding how I unwittingly maintained my problems and what more constructive alternative behaviours did I implement in achieving my goals? Are these problematic behaviours also a factor in my other problems and, if so, can I also apply the more constructive alternative behaviours that I developed in addressing my previous problems to these new problems?

Becoming Less Prone to Emotional Disturbance in the Future

If you want to become less prone to emotional disturbance in the future, you need to learn and apply general patterns of flexible and non-extreme thinking and constructive behaviour to a range of adversities that are likely to be troublesome for you. Seeking out such adversities, wherever possible and feasible, in a sensible way, while using these general patterns, is probably the best way of doing this. This is best implemented when the task at hand is difficult but not overwhelming for you. If you and your therapist have decided to work on helping you to become less prone to future emotional disturbance, the extent to which you agree on how you will approach this task is once again important.

Pursuing Healthy Self-Development

Have you ever wondered what the difference is between therapy and coaching? Well, one way of distinguishing the two is that therapy is more concerned with helping you overcome emotional problems, whereas coaching is focused on helping you to pursue goals that are related to healthy self-development. While the differences are, in fact, more blurred than this in reality, it is a useful rule of thumb when considering the differences between REBT and Rational Emotive Behavioural Coaching (REBC) for our purposes. Thus, when you are predominantly working with your therapist on matters largely concerned with promoting your healthy self-development, strictly speaking, you have moved into coaching and this needs to be acknowledged by both of you. Most organizations that offer non-fee-paying therapy do not regard coaching, by this definition, as part of their brief, and if you are paying your therapist a fee and getting reimbursed from a private health organization, be aware that it is unlikely that they will pay for coaching as opposed to therapy. However, if you are seeing a therapist privately, you are not seeking fee reimbursement and your therapist also has coaching as well as therapy skills, then REBC can be seen as a logical extension of successful REBT.

In the final chapter of this guide, I will discuss the situation where you, at the outset, choose to commit yourself to only one session.

Note

1 This schema can also be used with your main extreme and non-extreme attitude.

Chapter 9

When You Only Want to Commit to One Session

This Client Guide is based on what I call the conventional therapy mindset. This way of thinking about therapy sees the practice of therapy as stretching out over time with a beginning, a middle and an end, usually lasting for a good number of sessions. This is how most REBT therapists have been trained and it is the dominant viewpoint in the field of counselling and psychotherapy.

However, if you look at the attendance data at psychotherapy clinics across the world, you will discover something interesting – that the most frequent number of sessions that clients have at these clinics is one, followed by two, followed by three, etc. You might think that clients who attend one session of therapy must have been dissatisfied with the session and decided not to return. However, this is not the case. About 70%–80% of those who have one session are satisfied with that session. Furthermore, when clinics are organized such that incoming clients all have a single session of therapy on entry rather than an assessment session on entry, then 50% of those clients decide that they got what they wanted from the session and don't request any further sessions.

I included the present chapter in this book in case you, as a client, are only prepared to commit yourself to one session of REBT at the outset. If so, it is important that you are clear about this with your therapist. Not all REBT therapists are trained in single-session work and may think that they won't

DOI: 10.4324/9781003493198-10

be able to help you in one session. If so, ask them to refer you to an REBT therapist who can help you. Why might you wish to commit yourself to only one session of REBT, at least in the first instance?

First, you may have a problem for which you are seeking help and you think that you can be helped with that problem in one session with REBT.

Second, you may want a single session with an REBT therapist, not because you expect such a session to be all the help you need, but because you want guidance from the therapist concerning how you can tackle your nominated problem independently going forward. When I have an injury and seek help from a physiotherapist, I want that person to teach me what to do so I can practise these techniques on my own. I don't want to keep coming back to rehearse the techniques in the presence of the practitioner.

Third, you may seek a single session of REBT to discover whether this approach to therapy is right for you or not. Effectively, you are taking REBT for a test drive!

Finally, you may come for a single session seeking signposting help from the therapist concerning whether or not REBT will suit you and, if not, what therapeutic approach will suit you better. You don't expect your contact with the therapist to provide you with a solution to your problem in the session itself, but you want a pathway that you can follow where you can address your problems over time with a therapy or therapist that is right for you. You want the therapist to help you make that decision. You might choose to work with the REBT therapist you have consulted if you decide REBT is for you or you may decide to consult a different REBT therapist. Alternatively, if you decide that a different therapy approach would suit you better, then the therapist will refer you to a practitioner of that approach if they are able to.

If you have decided at the outset that you are only prepared to commit to a single session, it is important that you explain

to the therapist which of the above single-session therapy scenarios best represents the reason behind your decision. Having
said that, ideally, your therapist should ask you once they know
your decision to commit to one session in the first instance.

In the rest of this chapter, I will discuss the scenario where
you are seeking a single session for help with a specific issue
from the REBT therapist.

When You Want a Single REBT Session for Help with a Specific Problem

When you tell your therapist that you want them to help you in
a single session and they feel able to comply with that request,
they will use practical insights from what is called the single-
session therapy (SST) mindset as well as from REBT to help
you. An SST mindset is a way of thinking about therapy and the
practice that stems from that thinking that is based on the idea
that the therapist may only see the client once. In my experience, the fusion of practice from this mindset with REBT is a
particularly potent way of conducting a single session.

Prepare for the Session

If you have the opportunity to do so, it is a good idea to prepare
for the session. This will help you to get the most from the session. It is likely that your therapist will send you a pre-session
form inviting you to complete it to help you prepare and will
ask you to return it to them so that they can also prepare for the
session. If your therapist does not suggest that you complete
such a form, ask them for their advice on how you can best prepare for the session. Failing that, complete the form that I give
my SST clients to help them prepare for the session. I have
included this form in Appendix 4.
On the other hand, if you don't want to prepare for the session that is OK too. Such preparation should always be recommended by the therapist rather than mandated.

Give Your Informed Consent for Single-Session Therapy

As with other modes of helping, it is important that you give your informed consent for SST. To do that, you first need to be informed about what SST is. In my view:

> SST is a purposeful endeavour where both parties set out with the intention of helping the client in one session knowing that more help is available, if needed.

Once your therapist has informed you about SST, ask them any questions that you need answered before giving your consent.

It is also likely that your therapist will ask you for your permission for them to refer to your completed pre-session form (if you have completed and returned one) since doing so will not only save time but will help your therapist with their interventions.

At the Outset, Nominate a Problem and Agree a Focus with Your Therapist

Most people seeking SST will be looking for help to solve a specific problem, although this is not universally the case. Sometimes, the person may be looking to understand their problem better, for example. If this applies to you ask yourself the question, 'If I understood the issue better, what do I hope such understanding would lead to?' It is likely that you would hope that such understanding would lead to problem solution.

Given that, as I said earlier, most clients are looking for help from SST with a specific problem with which they have become stuck, I have assumed that this is the case for you and will proceed on that basis. Given this, it is vital that you agree with your therapist which one problem you are going to focus on (I call this the 'nominated problem'). This is important since you may have more than one problem you want help with.

Give Your Therapist Permission to Interrupt You, if Necessary

Once you and your therapist have agreed on a focus for the session (which will be your nominated problem) and you start to work on the problem with your therapist, be aware that your therapist may need to interrupt you to retain the agreed focus. This is because it is easy for you to wander away from the agreed focus and it is vital that you keep to this focus throughout the session if you are to get the most from it. Given this, before you start work on your nominated problem, it is likely that your therapist will give you a rationale for interrupting you, if necessary. Here is what I say to my SST clients on this point:

> Sometimes, I may need to interrupt you in order to keep us focused on the problem you want help with. This is because we may wander away from the focus, and it is important that I bring us back to it. May I have your permission to do this?

Once you have given your therapist permission for them to interrupt you, they will probably also ask you how best they can do so and then implement your chosen method if and when the need arises.

Negotiate with Your Therapist a Goal for the Session and for Your Nominated Problem

There are two sets of goals that are important to consider in REBT-informed SST: session goals and problem-related goals.

Session Goals

A session goal represents what you want and can realistically be expected to take away from the session that is relevant to your nominated problem. This is quite often a solution which you will develop with your therapist and need to implement after the session in order to address your nominated problem. In REBT-informed SST this solution will be a relevant flexible/non-extreme attitude that you will need to act on over time in order for it to help you achieve your problem-related goal.

Problem-Related Goals

A problem-related goal is what you seek to achieve in relation to your nominated problem so that the problem has been rendered a non-problem. As mentioned above, you need to implement the selected solution and do so over time to achieve your problem-related goal.

Figure 9.1 outlines the relationship between your nominated problem and your session-related and problem-related goals.

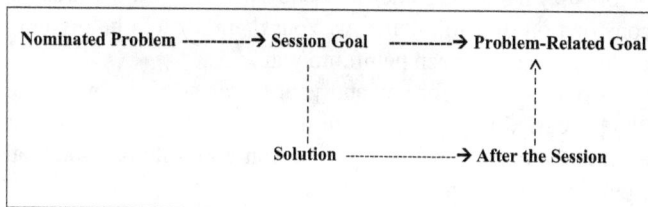

```
Nominated Problem ------------→ Session Goal   -----------→ Problem-Related Goal
                                     |                              ↑
                                     |                              |
                                     |                              |
                                     |                              |
                                  Solution  --------------------→ After the Session
```

Figure 9.1 The Relationship between Your Nominated Problem, and Your Session-Related and Problem-Related Goals

Note: This figure shows that your session goal will often be a solution to your nominated problem that you need to implement after the session so that you can achieve your problem-related goal. In REBT-informed SST this solution will most likely be a flexible/non-extreme attitude.

Making Sure You Are Still Talking about What Is Important to You

While keeping to the agreed focus is important in SST, your therapist will need to check periodically that you are still discussing an issue that is important to you. If not, and there is time, then it is important to change tack to something that is more of a priority to you. Having said that, if you and your therapist have taken time and care to help you select your nominated problem, then it is unlikely that you need to make this shift during the session.

What You Have Tried Before to Solve the Problem

You probably have tried a variety of strategies to help yourself with your nominated problem well before reaching out to seek professional help. While none of these strategies will have proven completely successful – for if they had, you would not be seeking therapeutic help now – some of what you have tried before may have had some value and can contribute towards the construction of a solution now. Your therapist will help you to build on what has been helpful to you.

Also, it is useful for you and your therapist to discover what you have tried in the past that hasn't proven helpful to you – or even made matters worse – so you can both rule out potential solutions that haven't helped you.

Discover and Potentially Make Use of Strategies You Have Successfully Used with Other Problems

It is also useful for you to discover if you have solved other emotionally related problems that may be different to your current nominated problem. If so, you may be able to apply strategies that have proven successful to you in other spheres to your current nominated problem. Your therapist will help you with this issue.

Identify and Utilize Your Internal and External Resources

Using the single-session mindset, your therapist will help you to look for both your internal and external resources so that you can make use of them at salient times during the session and afterwards.

Identify and Utilize Your Internal Resources

With respect to your internal resources, these tend to be tender-minded (e.g., compassion, empathy, kindness) or tough-minded (e.g., resilience, grit, assertion) and your therapist will either ask you about these directly (e.g., 'Which strengths do you have as a person that might help you in our work together on your nominated problem?') or they may discern these indirectly from what you have been discussing (e.g., 'Listening to you talk, it strikes me how resilient you have been in putting up with this situation for so long'). You can draw on your internal resources in developing a solution to your problem in the session or in applying the solution after the session. Also, if you have completed a pre-session form, you may have listed your strengths there which you can also consult.

Identify and Utilize Your External Resources

Your external resources may include (i) people in your life who can encourage you in your efforts to implement your selected solution, (ii) organizations that may offer you support and (iii) materials (e.g., therapeutic/educational that may aid you in solution implementation).

Using the REBT Perspective on Your Problem and Its Solution

You may not require any input from REBT to achieve your session goals. In such a case, you and your therapist can devise a solution that stems from the issues you have both covered and this can be done without reference to REBT. However, if what you have discussed with your therapist has not yielded potential solutions, then they will offer you their REBT 'take' on understanding your nominated problem and how it may be effectively addressed. Of course, when you have approached the therapist for single-session help precisely because they are an REBT therapist, then they will have used REBT from the outset together with the more general issues that I have discussed so far. I will discuss now how you and your therapist can efficiently use REBT within a single-session format.

Assessing the Problem Using the **ABC** Framework

When you nominate a problem to discuss in the single session, your therapist will ask you to select a specific example of this problem for you both to assess. A specific example means that the problem-related episode took place in a concrete situation with particular people present acting in identifiable ways. Such a specific example of the problem can be a recent example, a vivid example, a typical example or an anticipated example. The advantage of selecting an anticipated example is that once the example has been assessed and a solution developed then you can implement this solution in a similar future situation.

In using the *ABC* framework to assess your selected example, the most common order that your therapist will use is *CAB*. Thus, your therapist will begin by asking you what problematic unhealthy negative emotion (UNE) you experienced at *C*, together with how you acted and thought that went along with this emotion. Once you both have identified the major UNE, your therapist will use this to find the aspect of the situation that you were most disturbed about. This is the adversity at A.

Then, when you have identified both C and A, your therapist will use this information to identify your rigid/extreme attitude and the corresponding flexible/non-extreme attitude at B.

Examining Your Attitudes: Promoting Intellectual Insight

The heart of REBT is attitude change. This is the solution that REBT offers you in single-session work. There are two phases of such change: intellectual insight and emotional insight[1] (see Chapter 7). Intellectual insight, in this context, is achieved when you understand lightly and occasionally that your rigid and extreme attitudes are false, illogical and yield largely unconstructive results for you and that your alternative flexible and non-extreme attitudes are true, logical and yield largely constructive results for you. Intellectual insight is not sufficient for attitude change. Thus, it provides you with knowledge but does not impact significantly on your feelings and behaviour. When you have intellectual insight, you will say such things as 'I understand it in my head but don't feel it in my gut'. Your therapist will help you to achieve intellectual insight by encouraging you to examine both your rigid/extreme and flexible/non-extreme attitudes.

Putting Intellectual Insight into Practice: Towards Emotional Insight

By contrast, emotional insight, in this context, is achieved when you have a deeply held conviction that your rigid and extreme attitudes are false, illogical and yield largely unconstructive results for you and that your alternative flexible and non-extreme attitudes are true, logical and yield largely constructive results for you. Emotional insight is a sign that attitude change is underway. As such, having emotional insight does impact significantly on your feelings and behaviour. When you have emotional insight, you say such things as 'Not only do I understand it in my head, I also feel it in my gut'.

The best way that you can implement the attitude change solution that you and your therapist have selected is for you to put your intellectual insight into practice until it becomes emotional insight. This is done in the first instance by you developing an action plan with your therapist.

Develop an Action Plan and Commit Yourself to Implementing It[2]

The purpose of an action plan from an REBT perspective is to encourage you to take action in the face of your problem-related adversity that is consistent with your newly chosen flexible/non-extreme attitude and inconsistent with your currently held rigid/extreme attitude.

Elements of a Good Action Plan

As such, it should be remembered that results from a single session are achieved by what you do outside the session. Also, the achievement of your session goal represents the beginning of a process of change rather than the end of it, namely when you have reached your problem-related goal. Here are several features of a good action plan that should be considered by both you and your therapist as you work together to draw up such a plan.

TAKING RESPONSIBILITY

You need to take responsibility for implementing the plan. If you are not prepared to take ownership of implementing the action plan, then there is no point in your therapist helping you to develop the plan. Thus, before such work is undertaken, you need to state that you are prepared to do whatever you and your therapist agree should be a part of the action plan.

ENSURING THAT YOU CAN INTEGRATE THE SOLUTION INTO YOUR LIFE

You should be able to integrate the plan into your life. If you are not able to do this, you may begin to initiate the plan but quickly stop doing so because the effort required is, in your mind, too great. I am not suggesting here that you should only implement an action when it is easy for you to do so. What I am saying is that when it is part of your everyday routine, then you are more likely to implement the plan over time than when it is not part of your schedule. For example, it is not easy for a person with diabetes to inject themself with insulin several times a day, but if they make it part of their daily routine, then they will be able to maintain doing so.

CLARITY IS KEY

What you agree to do in your action plan needs to be clear. Therefore, the more specific the solution that is delineated in the plan, the better.

REMEMBERING THE PURPOSE OF THE SOLUTION

You need to see clearly how implementing the action plan can lead to the achievement of your problem-related goal. It will also help if you keep this connection at the forefront of your mind when implementing the solution in your everyday life.

The Components of a Good Action Plan

Perhaps the most important part of a solution-focused action plan is its components. These components are as follows:

- *What* you have agreed to do (i.e., the aspects of the solution).
- *When* you have agreed to implement the solution.

- *Where* the solution is to be implemented.
- *Whom* the solution is to be implemented with.
- *How often* the solution is to be implemented.

Make a Commitment to Implement the Action Plan

A commitment is a firm promise that you make with yourself to implement the action plan. It is *not* a commitment that you make to your therapist and, as such, you need to take them out of the equation. It may be that you have a doubt, reservation or objection to making such a commitment with yourself and, if so, it is important that you discuss this with your therapist. The outcome of the discussion is ideally that you make a firm commitment with yourself that you will implement the action plan.

IDENTIFYING AND DEALING WITH ANTICIPATED OBSTACLES

In addition to dealing with any doubts, reservations and objections you may have about committing yourself to implementing the action plan, it is also useful for you to identify potential obstacles to carrying it out. Your therapist will help you to do this and to help you to think about how you would respond should you encounter any obstacles that you anticipate.

MAKING A COMMITMENT PUBLIC OR KEEPING IT PRIVATE

When discussing making a commitment to implementing the action plan with your therapist, it is useful to think about whether there is value for you in making your commitment public or keeping it private. By making your commitment public, either generally or to certain people (e.g., those whom you regard as being among your external resources), you may experience a strengthened sense of resolve, which will help you implement your action plan. However, you may prefer to keep your commitment private. If you do, it is worthwhile thinking about the advantages and disadvantages of making your commitment part of a written contract with yourself. Your therapist will help you to work through these issues.

Ending the Session Well

Once you have made a commitment to implementing your agreed action plan, this is a reliable sign that the session is coming to an end. When this happens, your therapist will ask you to summarize the session.

Providing a Summary of the Session

There are two main reasons why it is better for you provide your own summary of the session than have your therapist summarize it for you. The first reason is that it keeps you actively involved in the session and encourages you to use your brain to summarize rather than borrow your therapist's brain for the purpose. The second reason is that you are more likely to take away what you regard as important from the session than what your therapist regards to be important. Thus, when your therapist asks you to provide your own summary, this encourages you to think about what for you were the highlights of the session. On the other hand, your therapist's summary would focus on what were the highlights for them, not you.

Ideally, your summary should include the nature of the nominated problem the two of you discussed, the solution you came up with to address the problem, and the action plan you agreed which you have given your commitment to implement.

Specify Your Takeaways

In SST, your takeaway is what you have learned from the session that, in your mind, is worth taking away from the session. You may have covered this in your summary, or you may disclose it once you have been asked for it by your therapist. Don't try and take away too much from the session. One or two takeaways that you deem to be important and which you think will make a significant difference to your life going forward are enough. Trying to take away any more may confuse or overwhelm you.

Ideally, then, you should leave the session with a solution, an action plan and new learning derived from your conversation with your therapist.

Think about How to Generalize the Solution and/or Your Takeaways

If feasible, your therapist should ask you if you can see ways of generalizing (a) the solution that you have developed with them and (b) your takeaways to other relevant aspects of your life that you haven't discussed with your therapist, For example, if your therapist has helped you to develop a good solution to dealing with criticism at work, think about whether you can use the solution in other settings where you may face criticism. Also, think about whether what you have learned is applicable to other adversities that you struggle with that you have not had an opportunity to discuss.

In general, most clients need help to generalize what they learn from therapy sessions and if your therapist does not provide you with such an opportunity, you may not think of doing so yourself.

Leaving the Session Satisfied that You Have Had a Final Opportunity to Make Comments or Ask Questions

It is important that the session has a good ending and, as such, your therapist should give you a last opportunity to tell them something that you would regret not telling them or to ask them something that you would regret not asking. In having this final chance, use it to say or ask something that is relevant to what you have covered with your therapist in the session. Don't use it to bring up a new problem in the closing moments of the session.

Agreeing the Way Forward

You will recall from my definition of SST that having the session does not preclude you from accessing further help. Having said this, SST does provide an opportunity for you to leave the session with what you have come for. Most SST practitioners consider that it is important for clients to have an opportunity to reflect on what they have learned, digest their learning and implement their action plan to see how they get on before making a decision concerning whether or not to seek further help. Thus, it is not a good idea in general for your therapist to offer you an opportunity at the end of the session to make an appointment for a further session. There will, of course, be exceptions to this. Thus, what you have discussed with your therapist may have evoked strong feelings in you that may not have been resolved at the end of the session, and you both consider that harm would befall you if a further session is not arranged before you leave.

However, it is generally a good idea for you to have an opportunity to get the most from the session and this is done by you having time to put into practice what you have learned from the session and to see what happens. At that point, you may decide you don't need further help or you may decide that you do. The choice is up to you.

We have now come to the end of this Client Guide. I hope you have found it useful and that it has given you some ideas concerning how to get the most out of REBT. I would appreciate receiving any feedback that might improve this guide based on your experiences of using it. Please email me at windy@windy-dryden.com

Notes

1 I will discuss emotional insight below.
2 This section is relevant whether you have selected an REBT-informed solution or one not informed by REBT.

Appendix 1

What Is REBT?

There are a number of approaches to therapy and it is important that you understand something of the one that I practise which is known as Rational Emotive Behaviour Therapy (REBT). REBT is based on an old idea attributed to Epictetus, a Roman philosopher, who said that 'Men are disturbed not by things, but by their views of things'. In REBT, we have modified this and say: 'People are not disturbed by the adversities that they face. Rather, they disturb themselves about these adversities by the rigid and extreme attitudes that they hold towards them.' Once they have disturbed themselves they try to get rid of their disturbed feelings in ways that ultimately serve to maintain their problems.

As an REBT therapist I will help you to identify, examine and change the rigid and extreme attitudes that we argue underpin your emotional problems and to develop alternative flexible and non-extreme attitudes. I will also help you to examine the ways in which you have tried to help yourself that haven't worked and encourage you to develop and practise more effective, longer-lasting strategies. At the beginning of therapy, we will consider your problems one at a time and I will teach you a framework which will help you to break down your problems into their constituent parts. I will also teach you a variety of methods for examining and changing your rigid and extreme attitudes and a variety of methods to help you to consolidate and strengthen your alternative flexible and non-extreme attitudes. As therapy proceeds, I will help you to take increasing responsibility for using these methods and my ultimate aim is to help you to become your own therapist. As this happens, we will meet less frequently until you feel you can cope on your own.

Therapeutic Contract with Windy Dryden

1. Length of therapy sessions

   Therapy sessions are 50 minutes in length unless otherwise agreed. They will be face-to-face or by Zoom. If the latter, I will provide you with a link the day before the session.

2. Fee

   My fee is £… per session pro rata. The method of payment is by mutual agreement. I will give you two months' notice of any increase to my fee.

   Please note that as your contract is with me, I expect you to pay me directly. I do not invoice insurance companies, but will provide you with receipts for you to claim reimbursement from them.

3. Cancellation policy

   My cancellation policy is as follows. In order for you to cancel a session without charge you need to give me 48 hours' notice. My full fee will be levied if notice within this period is not given. An exception to this is if you, or a member of your immediate family, suffer a sudden serious illness.

   If I cancel a session, I will give you 48 hours' notice. If I do not do so, then your next therapy session will be free of charge. An exception to this is if I, or a member of my immediate family, suffer a sudden serious illness.

4. Confidentiality policy
   My confidentiality policy is as follows. All sessions are confidential with the following exceptions:

   - If you pose a serious threat to your own life or well-being and are not prepared to take steps to protect yourself, I will take steps to provide such protection.
   - If you pose a serious threat to the life or well-being of another person and are not prepared to take steps to protect them, I will take steps to provide such protection.
   - If I am legally mandated to make my notes available.
   - If my fees are not paid and I take legal recourse to recover these fees.
   - If you wish me to provide information about our sessions to a third party, I require notification of this request in writing.

5. My working environment

   - As I do not have waiting room facilities, I would be grateful if you would ring my bell at your appointed appointment time and not before.
   - Please do not attend a therapy session if you are intoxicated or are under the influence of a mind-altering drug.
   - Also, as the smell of cigarette smoke lingers and may affect other clients whom I may see after your session, I respectfully request that you do not smoke an hour before your session.
   - If we are meeting by Zoom, please ensure that you are on your own in a professional working space with good Wi-Fi.

I have read, understood and agree with the above points.
Signature of client.............. Signature of therapist.................
Print name......................... Print name ....
Date................................ Date ....

Possible Reasons for Not Completing Homework (Self-Help) Tasks

Name............... Date..........

The following is a list of reasons that various clients have given for not doing their homework (self-help) tasks during the course of REBT. Because the speed of improvement depends primarily on the number of such tasks that you are willing to do, it is of great importance to pinpoint any reasons that you may have for not doing this work. It is important to look for these reasons at the time that you feel a reluctance to do your task or a desire to put off doing it. Hence, it is best to fill out this questionnaire at that time. If you have any difficulty filling out this form and returning it to your therapist, it might be best to do it together during a therapy session.

Rate each statement by ringing 'T' (True) or 'F' (False). 'T' indicates that you agree with it; 'F' means the statement does not apply at this time.

1. It seems that nothing can help me, so there is no point in trying.   T/F
2. It wasn't clear, I didn't understand what I had to do.   T/F
3. I thought that the particular method my therapist had suggested would not be helpful. I didn't really see the value of it.   T/F
4. It seemed too hard.   T/F
5. I am willing to do self-help tasks, but I keep forgetting. T/F
6. I did not have enough time. I was too busy.   T/F

7. If I do something my therapist suggests I do, it's not as good as if I come up with my own ideas.   T/F
8. I don't really believe I can do anything to help myself.   T/F
9. I have the impression my therapist is trying to boss me around or control me.   T/F
10. I worry about my therapist's disapproval. I believe that what I do just won't be good enough for them.   T/F
11. I felt too bad, sad, nervous, upset (underline the appropriate word[s]) to do it.   T/F
12. It would have upset me to do the homework.   T/F
13. It was too much to do.   T/F
14. It's too much like going back to school again.   T/F
15. It seemed to be mainly for my therapist's benefit.   T/F
16. Homework or self-help tasks have no place in therapy.   T/F
17. Because of the progress I've made, these tasks are likely to be of no further benefit to me.   T/F
18. Because these tasks have not been helpful in the past, I couldn't see the point of doing this one.   T/F
19. I don't agree with this particular approach to therapy.   T/F
20. OTHER REASONS (please write them):

Pre-Session Form

I invite you to fill in this form before your session with me. This will help you to prepare for the session so that you can get the most from it. It also helps me to help you as effectively as I can. Please return it by email attachment before our session. Please be brief and concise in your answers.

Name: .... Date: ....

1. **What is the issue that you want to focus on in the session?**
   Be concise. In one or two sentences get to the heart of the problem, if possible.

2. **Why is this significant?**
   What's at stake? How does this affect your life? What is the future impact if the issue is not resolved?

3. **What is your goal in discussing this issue in the session?**
   What are the specific results you would like to achieve by
   the end of the <u>session</u> that would give you the sense that you
   have begun to make progress on the issue?

4. **Specify briefly the relevant background information.**
   What do you think I need to know about the issue to help
   you with it? Summarize in bullet points.

5. **How have you tried to deal with the issue up to this point?**
   What steps, successful or unsuccessful, have you taken so
   far in addressing the issue?

6. **What are the strengths or inner resources that you have as a person that you could draw upon while tackling the issue?**

   If you struggle with answering this question, think of what people who really know you and who are on your side would say.

7. **Who are the people in your life who can support you as you tackle the issue?**

   Name them and say what help each can provide.

8. **What help do you hope I can best provide you in the session? Please check the main <u>one</u> only. Do not check more than one box.**

   □ Help me to develop greater understanding of the issue

   □ Help me by just listening while I talk about the issue

   □ Help me to express my feelings about the issue

   □ Help me to solve an emotional or behavioural problem; help me get unstuck

□ Help me to make a decision

□ Help me to resolve a dilemma

□ Help me by signposting me to the most appropriate
   service for my situation

□ Other (please specify):

Thank you.
Windy Dryden

Index

Neff, Kristin 76
nominated problems *see*
    problems/nominated problems

obstacles to change 41, 52–67;
    dealing with 62–67; due to
    client factors 28, 56–59; due
    to therapist factors 59–62; due
    to working alliance problems
    52–55

past experiences 7–8, 24–25, 54
personal issues, therapist's
    61–62
practical agreements 11–18;
    cancellation policies 14–15,
    17, 100; confidentiality
    policies 16–17, 101; fees
    12–15, 100; form of the
    contract 17–18, 100–101;
    frequency of sessions 16;
    length of sessions 12, 100;
    total number of sessions 13,
    15–16
practical problems 21
pre-session forms 84, 104–107
preparation for sessions 31–34;
    goal lists 32; matters arising
    34; pre-session forms 84,
    104–107; preparing what to
    discuss 32–33; problem lists
    31–32; session agendas 33–34
primary problems 36
problem-based approach 37
problem lists 20–21, 31–32
problem-related goals 87
problems/nominated problems:
    admitting you have a problem
    35–36; agreements about
    20–21; assessment of
    36–37, 69–71, 90–91;
    case formulation 36–37;

disagreements about 53–54;
    focusing on one at a time
    37–38; meta-problems 36;
    past experiences and 7–8,
    24–25, 54; practical problems
    21; primary problems 36;
    selecting nominated problem
    33, 85; short-term 'solutions'
    to 56–57; specific examples of
    33, 38; unwitting maintenance
    of 7–8, 24–25
process of change 35–41
progress, lack of 52–67; dealing
    with 62–67; due to client
    factors 28, 56–59; due to
    therapist factors 59–62; due
    to working alliance problems
    52–55
psychotherapeutic approaches,
    common factors 3–5

Rational Emotive Behaviour
    Coaching (REBC) 80
Rational Emotive Behaviour
    Therapy (REBT): *ABC*
    framework 33, 90–91; brief
    description of 10, 98–99;
    deciding if REBT is right for
    you 3–10; distinctive features
    5–10; using in single-session
    therapy 90–92
rehearsing: homework tasks 48;
    imagery 77
relapse prevention skills 77–78
relapsing 40
review sessions 30
rigid and extreme attitudes 7, 8, 24,
    38–39, 71–72, 91, 92, 98–99
roles *see* client role; therapist role

safety behaviours 7
self-acceptance, unconditional 76

For Product Safety Concerns and Information please contact our EU
representative GPSR@taylorandfrancis.com
Taylor & Francis Verlag GmbH, Kaufingerstraße 24, 80331 München, Germany

www.ingramcontent.com/pod-product-compliance
Lightning Source LLC
Chambersburg PA
CBHW070350270326
41926CB00017B/4077